The Nuts and
Bolts of
Cardiac Pacing

Commissioning Editor: Gina Almond
Editorial Assistant: Jamie Hartman-Boyce
Development Editor: Beckie Brand and Kate Newell

The Nuts and Bolts of Cardiac Pacing

2ND EDITION

Tom Kenny

Vice President Academic Affairs
St Jude Medical, Austin, Texas

WILEY-BLACKWELL

A John Wiley & Sons, Ltd., Publication

This edition first published 2008, © 2005, 2008 St Jude Medical

Blackwell Publishing was acquired by John Wiley & Sons in February 2007. Blackwell's publishing program has been merged with Wiley's global Scientific, Technical and Medical business to form Wiley-Blackwell.

Registered office: John Wiley & Sons Ltd, The Atrium, Southern Gate, Chichester, West Sussex, PO19 8SQ, United Kingdom

Editorial office: Blackwell Publishing Ltd, 9600 Garsington Road, Oxford, OX4 2DQ, United Kingdom

For details of our global editorial offices, for customer services and for information about how to apply for permission to reuse the copyright material in this book please see our website at www.wiley.com/wiley-blackwell

Library of Congress Cataloguing-in-Publication Data

Kenny, Tom, 1954-
  The nuts and bolts of cardiac pacing / Tom Kenny. -- 2nd ed.
    p. ; cm.
  Includes bibliographical references and index.
  ISBN 978-1-4051-8403-8 (alk. paper)
  1. Cardiac pacing. I. Title.
  [DNLM: 1. Cardiac Pacing, Artificial. 2. Pacemaker, Artificial. WG 168 K36n 2008]
  RC684.P3K465 2008
  617.4'120645--dc22

                                                                                    2008002785

ISBN: 978-1-4051-8403-8

A catalogue record for this book is available from the British Library.

Set in 9.5/12 pt Minion by Sparks, Oxford – www.sparkspublishing.com

First edition published 2005
Second edition 2008

5   2014

Contents

Introduction

This book was first published in 2005, but the idea for this book dates back at least 10 years earlier. I was a former clinician who had just taken a job with a pacemaker manufacturer so I could educate clinicians about pacemakers. I realized pretty quickly that there was no book for the kind of classes I was starting to teach.

That is not to say that there are not fine books on cardiac pacing. There are many excellent books available, but they tend to be written by pacing gurus for other pacing gurus.

I did not start out wanting to write books – in fact, I tried pretty hard over the years to avoid it – but it seemed to me that this was the book that so many clinicians needed. It was also the one book I needed for my courses that simply could not be found on the market.

Back when I was in the clinic, you learned about pacing only if you absolutely had to know it and you could find somebody to help mentor you. In my background, I learned from Dr Orlando Maytin, Dr Michael Chizner, Barbara Perra, Kathy King, and Eliot Ostrow. These people took plenty of time to educate me in the fine points of cardiac pacing. I owe them a great debt.

In today's hectic clinical environment, many clinicians tasked with managing device patients may not enjoy the luxury of having qualified, willing, and generous mentors to teach them. Most device manufacturers offer excellent training programs to those clinicians who can carve some precious time out of their already jam-packed schedules to participate.

In short, it is more likely than ever that today's clinical personnel have to know pacing and it is less likely than ever that they will find mentors or the time.

That is why I wrote this book. It was intended to be a book on pacing for clinicians who were educated in clinical practice but not necessarily knowledgeable about pacemakers. The book was such a tremendous success that I was grateful for the opportunity this year to go back and update it.

A lot has changed in pacing in even the few years since this book was first published. The DAVID trial, for one thing, has changed the way a lot of people think about pacing. New device features and software have been added.

Yet the basics of pacing are still the same.

If you are a clinician who sees pacemaker patients and feels overwhelmed by pacing technology or if you are a busy clinician who just needs to know more about the pacemaker patients all around you (they're everywhere!), this book was written for you. I hope that pacing experts and novices alike can derive benefit from this book, but my heart has always been with the rookie.

If you are new to the world of pacing, welcome aboard! These tiny but powerful medical devices have literally given millions of people around the world a new lease of life. As they grow more technologically advanced, they also become easier to use – providing you know the basics. This book will introduce you to what pacemakers can do and how they work. There is a lot to learn, so be patient, but it is not really very difficult when you approach it systematically.

As always, I welcome your comments and ideas on this book.

Tom Kenny
Austin, January 2008

CHAPTER 1

The healthy heart

The human heart – about the size of a clenched fist – is the center of a complex system designed to help the body nourish its organs with life-giving oxygen and to remove waste products in the form of carbon dioxide from the body. Simple animals, such as insects, have an open circulatory system, in which the heart pumps blood through the body cavity, washing the organs directly. More complex animals, including all vertebrates, have a closed circulatory system, which requires the heart to pump blood throughout a network of vessels. No system of vessels is as complex as that of a human being, and it is so closely related to the heart's function that we frequently talk of the "cardiovascular" or CV system rather than the heart in isolation.

In the human CV system, blood stays in the vessels while oxygen and carbon dioxide are exchanged by diffusion through the vessel walls. So intricate is the human circulatory system that there are actually two complementary networks: a pulmonary circulatory system, designed to get deoxygenated blood to the lungs so it can be "revitalized" with oxygen, and a systemic circulatory system which pumps oxygen-rich blood throughout the body to nourish muscles, tissues, and organs.

At the heart of this elaborate circulatory system is, literally, the heart. At its most basic, the healthy human heart is an efficient and effective pump, beating about 70 times a minute without stopping over the course of a human lifespan. The circulatory system is designed to get oxygen-rich blood where it is needed when it is needed, so the heart regulates its own activities, beating more rapidly during times of increased oxygen consumption and more slowly during periods of decreased demand, such as rest and sleep.

The heart is a muscle with four hollow chambers: two upper and two lower (Fig. 1.1). On top are the atria (singular: atrium), thin-walled, small chambers that take their name from our architec-

tural word "atrium." They are the ante-chambers or front lobby of the heart. The two lower chambers are large, thick-walled, heavily muscled chambers called ventricles. The ventricles are responsible for most of the pumping action of the heart.

While physicians can talk about the heart in terms of atria and ventricles, or upper and lower chambers, it is also possible to talk about the heart in terms of right side and left side. The right side of the

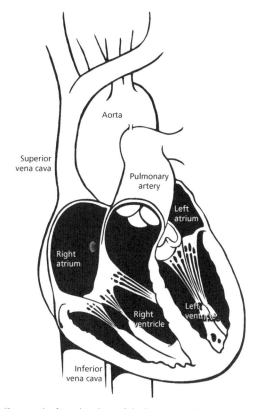

Fig. 1.1 The four chambers of the heart with the largest vessels in the body: the superior and inferior vena cava (which feed deoxygenated blood to the heart) and the aorta (which carries oxygen-rich blood from the heart to the rest of the body).

The Nuts and Bolts of Cardiac Pacing, 2nd edition. By Tom Kenny. © 2008 St Jude Medical, ISBN: 978-1-4501-8403-8.

heart consists of the right atrium and the right ventricle, which are connected to each other through the tricuspid valve. When deoxygenated blood flows back to the heart to become reoxygenated, it first enters the right side of the heart. This deoxygenated blood arrives at the right side of the heart through the body's largest veins: the superior vena cava and the inferior vena cava. (In this case, "superior" and "inferior" refer to physical locations of "above" and "below" the heart.) The right side of the heart pumps this oxygen-depleted blood back out through the pulmonary artery to the lungs, where it picks up much-needed oxygen. Once the blood has received oxygen, the venous system routes the blood back into the heart, this time to the left side.

Loaded with oxygen, the blood reenters the heart through the pulmonary veins into the left atrium and the left ventricle, connected by the mitral valve. The left side of the heart pumps the blood back out to the rest of the body (the systemic circulatory system) through the aorta and the arteries that branch off the aorta.

Cardiac pacing and defibrillation leads for conventional pacemaker and implantable cardioverter defibrillator (ICD) systems are implanted in the right side of the heart. A transvenous lead – i.e. a wire that goes through a patient's vein – can "go with the flow" of blood into the right atrium, through the tricuspid valve, and into the right ventricle. Conventional pacemakers and ICDs have found that pacing the right side of the heart is sufficient to cause a contraction of the entire heart. More recent cardiac resynchronization therapy (CRT) devices require a pacing lead to be implanted in both the right and the left sides of the heart. This poses some technical challenges as a transvenous lead cannot readily travel to this area without going through the heart and then *against* the heart's natural powerful pumping action. CRT therapy and lead placement falls outside the scope of this book, but it is mentioned to give the reader a more complete view of the therapies available.

Myocardial cells

The heart pumps blood through rhythmic contractions or beats, also known as "depolarizations." Depolarization explains what happens to the heart at the cellular level, which is the best way to understand

how it beats. Unlike other muscles, which respond to the control of the brain, the heart regulates its own actions without specific input from the brain. To accomplish this, it relies on some of the body's most complex cellular constructions and interactions.

The healthy human heart has two main types of cells: myocardial cells (heart muscle cells) and conduction system cells (electrical cells). Myocardial cells are the ones that make the heart beat.

All heart cells are cylindrical and branch at their ends into one or more limbs. These cardiac cells are held together with intercalated disks sandwiched between them to form a network (Fig. 1.2). Think of myocardial cells as a dense forest of trunks and limbs and branches with intercalated disks forming connections. These intercalated disks help conduct electricity from cell to cell by relaying the impulse.

While myocardial cells do not conduct electricity as rapidly as the electrical cells of the heart, they do have the property of contractility, an ability to shorten and then return to their original length. Contractility allows myocardial cells to stretch and snap back into place. In this way, the myocardium

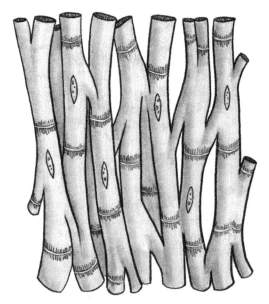

Fig. 1.2 Myocardial cells are specialized cylindrical cells that relax and contract, changing the shape of the heart. Intercalated disks are membranes that include gap junctions for conducting electricity rapidly from one cell to another.

Table 1.1 Common cardiac drugs

	Increases myocardial contractility	Decreases myocardial contractility
Sympathomimetics (digitalis, bretylium)	X	
Beta blockers		X
Quinidine		X
Procainamide		X
Excessive potassium		X
Hypovolemia	X	
Anemia	X	
Hypocalcemia		X
Hypothyroidism		X
Emotion	X	
Increased venous return to the heart	X	
Shock		X
Fever	X	
Exercise	X	
Emotion	X	

or heart muscle is able to expand to take in blood and then to contract powerfully to pump the blood back out.

Myocardial contractility responds to a variety of influences. Physical stimuli (including exercise, emotion, fever) and some drugs (sympathomimetics such as digitalis) can increase myocardial contractility, forcing the heart to beat more vigorously. Likewise, other stimuli (shock, hypothyroidism, and others) and some drugs (beta blockers, quinidine, procainamide, and excess potassium) can decrease myocardial contractility (Table 1.1).

The heartbeat

An electrical impulse traveling through the heart causes the cardiac cells to depolarize and contract. The human heartbeat is not one single contraction, but is a precisely timed sequence of four specific events (Fig. 1.3).

Starting with the heart at rest, blood flows naturally into the heart. The valves are open and the heart gets a considerable amount of blood into it through a descriptively named process known as the passive filling of the ventricles. The atria are relaxed in a state known as atrial diastole. When an electrical impulse fires in the heart, the heart beat begins its four-part cycle.

The atria contract (atrial systole) while the ventricles remain relaxed (ventricular diastole). Since the ventricles are already passively filled with blood, this atrial contraction forces even more blood into the ventricles. Known as the atrial contribution to ventricle filling (or "atrial kick") this atrial contraction ensures that the ventricles are filled to the point where they have to stretch to accommodate all of the blood within them. The valves joining atrial to ventricular chambers close, so the ventricles now contain a great deal of blood that cannot backflow into the atria.

There is a brief period of rest – measured in ms (thousandths of a second).

The ventricular cells depolarize forcing a contraction of the powerful ventricular muscles (ventricular systole). This forces blood out over the pulmonary artery (and into the lungs) on the right side or into the aorta (and into the systemic circulatory system) on the left side. This beat is the most powerful action of the heart and it forms the largest complex on an electrocardiogram (ECG).

After contraction, the ventricular muscles repolarize or resume their resting state. The heart resumes the cycle with the passive filling of the ventricles.

Seen on an ECG, a healthy heartbeat shows three distinct wave patterns plus some flat areas of rest (Fig. 1.4). The cycle begins with an atrial beat, shown by the small P wave on the ECG. The flat line between the P wave and the next complex indicates the short rest phase. The large complex, called the

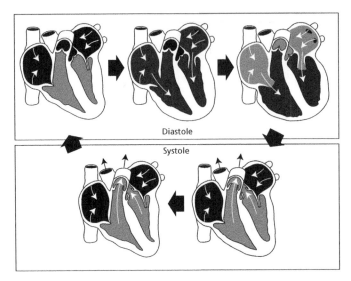

Diastole

Systole

Fig. 1.3 The heartbeat is a sequence of events that begins with ventricular diastole when the ventricles relax, begin to fill, and complete filling. The next phase is ventricular systole when the ventricles contract and empty. Atrial systole helps completely fill the ventricles, and the valves work to ensure that blood moves efficiently through the heart.

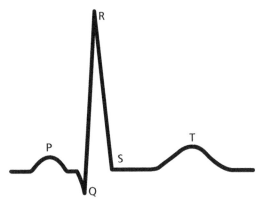

Fig. 1.4 The main waveforms on a surface ECG correspond to the various parts of the heartbeat. The P wave indicates atrial depolarization. This is followed after a short delay by the large QRS complex, which represents ventricular depolarization. A short pause follows, then the ventricles repolarize. This is shown on an ECG by the T wave. The ventricular contraction is the "biggest" event in the cardiac cycle in terms of creating electrical energy, so it appears as the largest portion of the ECG.

QRS complex, is the ECG depiction of the ventricular contraction. As the ventricles are massively large compared to the atria, the ventricular complex dominates the ECG in terms of size. There are three strokes to the ventricular complex, known as the Q, R, and S. Taken together, they describe the ventricular contraction. Another short expanse of flat line shows a rest period. The last wave in the complex is a T wave, which is the electrical depiction of the ventricles repolarizing or resuming their old form.

The pump

The healthy heart beats in a four-part cycle consisting of systole (contraction) and diastole (rest) of upper and lower chambers. When the cycles are precisely timed, the heart is able to pump very effectively. The passive filling of the ventricles combined with the "atrial kick" assure that the maximum amount of blood is brought into the ventricles to be pumped back out. The ventricles – forced to stretch to accommodate the large quantity of blood – contract even more strongly because of this stretch (Starling's law of contractility states that the heart muscle is like a rubber band; the more it is stretched, the more force with which it will snap back). In good working order, the valves in the heart (tricuspid, mitral, pulmonary, and aortic) open clearly and close securely, thus allowing and stopping the flow of blood at the right moments.

The healthy heart relies on a system of vessels to transport blood in and out of the heart. In addition, a separate network of very fine vessels delivers oxygenated blood to the heart muscle itself: the coronary arteries are the heart's own system for nourishment. When these small vessels get clogged or damaged in coronary artery disease (CAD), the heart muscle may be deprived of the oxygen it needs to work properly.

The healthy heart is able to keep a large amount of blood in constant circulation in the body. When the body consumes more oxygen, the heart increases its pumping action to keep pace, usually by beating faster. In its perfect state, the heart does a remarkable job of keeping the body fueled with oxygen and exchanging waste products. Of course, many things can occur in such a complex system to impair its ability to perform. Some of the main malfunctions of the cardiovascular system – the heart and its vessels – are listed below.

• **Coronary artery disease** in which the network of small arteries that help feed the heart muscle itself become occluded, typically through hyperlipidemia (cholesterol and plaque deposits). This can limit the heart's ability to perform. In extreme cases, blood flow is blocked causing a heart attack and ischemia to portions of the heart muscle itself. A coronary artery bypass graft (CABG) procedure is a typical intervention to treat blocked coronary arteries.

• **Heart failure** refers to the gradual decline in the ability of the heart muscle to pump efficiently. Although there are many manifestations of heart failure, all involve a deterioration of the pumping capacity of the heart. In some cases, the heart muscle gets flabby and enlarged; this is known as dilated cardiomyopathy. In other cases, such as hypertrophic cardiomyopathy, the ventricular wall thickens to the point that not only can it not contract properly, it cannot hold an adequate quantity of blood for a heartbeat. Heart failure is typically treated with drugs, but biventricular device therapy (sometimes called cardiac resynchronization therapy or CRT) holds enormous promise, at least for certain types of patients.

• **Conduction disorders** occur when the electrical system that governs the heart does not work correctly. In such cases, the heart muscle may still be strong, but the electrical signals do not allow the heart to function properly. Conduction disorders, also known as rhythm disorders, are the subject of the next chapter – and the main heart condition treated by pacemakers.

Further reading

Huszar RJ. *Basic Dysrhythmias: Interpretation and Management*. St Louis, MO: C. V. Mosby, 1988.

The nuts and bolts of the healthy heart

• The human heart is a four-chambered pump that circulates blood through a complex network of vessels.

• The heart can be talked about in terms of upper chambers (atria) and lower chambers (ventricles) or right side (right atrium and right ventricle) and left side (left atrium and left ventricle). The right side pumps oxygen-depleted blood through the pulmonary artery over the lungs, while the left side receives the oxygenated blood and pumps it out through the aorta and into the rest of the body.

• It is much easier to implant a pacing lead in the right side of the heart (which is needed for conventional pacemakers) than the left side of the heart (which is required for "biventricular pacing").

• When the heart "beats," it contracts owing to changes at the cellular level called "depolarizations."

• The heart has two types of cells: myocardial cells (which can depolarize) and conduction system cells (which conduct electricity).

• Myocardial contractility (how the heart muscle contracts) responds to many influences, including exercise, drugs, and fever.

• A single heartbeat breaks down into four phases: (a) atrial systole, when the atria contract but the ventricles remain relaxed; (b) rest; (c) ventricular systole, when the blood is pumped out over the body as the atria relax; (d) rest.

• An ECG is a visual depiction of the heartbeat taken from electricity on the surface of the skin. The P wave is the atrial activity. It is followed by the large QRS complex, which represents ventricular depolarization. The T wave after the QRS represents ventricular repolarization or the resumption of the resting state.

• Systole is the contraction phase, and diastole is the resting phase. Thus systolic blood pressure is

Continued p.6

Continued.

the blood pressure that occurs when the heart is pumping. Diastolic blood pressure is the blood pressure that occurs when the heart is at rest.

• Coronary artery disease (CAD) occurs when the network of tiny vessels that feed the heart muscle become occluded and limit the heart's ability to perform.

• Heart failure is the gradual decline in the ability of the heart muscle to pump efficiently.

Heart failure may manifest itself as a flabby, enlarged heart (dilated cardiomyopathy) or as the abnormal thickening of the ventricular wall (hypertrophic cardiomyopathy).

• Conduction disorders occur when the heart's electrical system does not work properly. Pacemakers address conduction disorders of the heart.

CHAPTER 2

The conduction system

Although we can think of the heart as a pump and the cardiovascular system as a "plumbing system," the heart is also regulated by an elaborate electrical network known as the "conduction system." The heart has unique electrical properties that make it different from any other muscle in the human body. To understand the electrical system of the heart, it is necessary to get down to the cellular level.

All cardiac cells have the ability to conduct electrical impulses. In terms of structure, cardiac cells are cylindrical and branch into two or more limbs at either end. Cardiac cells connect with other cardiac cells at the end of these branches through a type of cellular membrane called an "intercalated disk" (Fig. 2.1). These intercalated disks – found nowhere else in the body – sandwich themselves between the cylindrical cardiac cells. With its profusion of branches and sandwiched disks, cardiac cells form an almost tree-like network.

Electricity can travel through any part of the body, but nowhere else in the body is the pathway for electrical energy as efficient and specific as in the heart. When an electrical pulse enters the cardiac system, it travels rapidly from cell to cell by jumping through the intercalated disks. These intercalated disks facilitate and speed the flow of electrical energy so that an electrical impulse that enters the heart moves swiftly through cardiac tissue. Clinicians sometimes call these intercalated disks "gap junctions" because they join (junction) the spaces (gaps) between cardiac cells in such a way that allows electricity to flow smoothly and very rapidly.

The heart contains two types of cells: myocardial cells (muscle cells responsible for contracting and relaxing to make the heart pump) and electrical cells. Both conduct electricity efficiently, but the electrical cells of the heart have far more intercalated disks and can conduct electricity up to six times faster than myocardial cells. These electrical cells form the pathways for electricity through the heart. In the healthy heart, they allow for the proper timing of all phases of the human heartbeat.

The electrical pathway

These electrical cells form an electrical pathway through the heart which can be considered the heart's conduction system. It begins with a small collection of highly specialized cells known as the sinoatrial (SA) node, located on the high right atrium. The SA node contains a special type of cardiac electrical cell with the property of automaticity. This means these cells have the ability to spontaneously generate electricity.

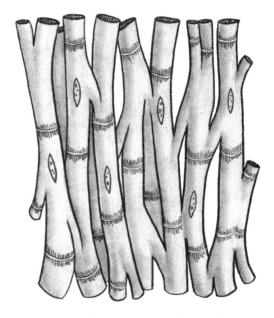

Fig. 2.1 Cardiac cells consist of myocardial cells and specialized electrical cells. Intercalated disks act as "gap junctions" to facilitate and speed up the flow of electricity. In fact, electricity can travel through a gap junction six times faster than it can travel through the myocardial cells.

When working properly, the SA node fires precisely timed electrical output pulses that flow through the conduction system and keep the heart beating properly. The SA node does not require intervention by the brain to know when and how to fire; it happens automatically. For this reason, the cells of the SA node are also called "pacemaker cells" and make up the heart's natural pacemaker. An implantable pacemaker is used when some part of the heart's conduction system fails and an external pacemaker is needed to help the heart beat at the right pace.

The electrical pulse that causes a heartbeat is issued from the SA node. It then travels along a special pathway through the atria down to the atrioventricular (AV) node. The AV node is another group of highly specialized cardiac electrical cells. Located on the right side of the interatrial septum near the opening of the coronary sinus, the AV node acts like a relay station. The electrical energy flows to the AV node where it is delayed for a short time and then allowed to travel down into the ventricles. This AV nodal timing delay is measured in split seconds (ms or thousandths of a second), but this fraction of a second allows the atria to contract and relax prior to the ventricular contraction.

From the AV node, the electrical energy then flows downward through the ventricles along the bundle of His, the right and left bundle branches, and the Purkinje network. These various components are sometimes grouped together and called the His–Purkinje system. The bundle of His is uppermost, and it links the AV node with the right and left branches. The right and left branches – as the name implies – carry the electrical energy to the right and left ventricles. The right and left branches run down the middle of the heart, along the right and left sides of the ventricular septum. As they travel down into the ventricles, the branches get smaller and smaller and form an increasing number of limbs until they become the very fine network of Purkinje fibers that conduct electricity throughout all parts of the myocardium (Fig. 2.2).

As electricity travels through the heart, it causes the myocardial cells (which conduct electricity, but

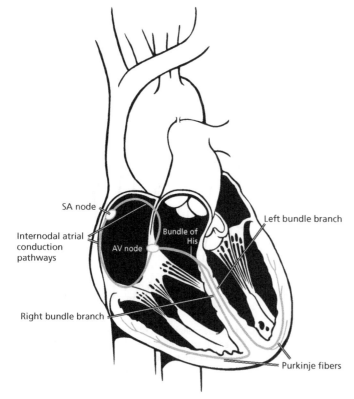

SA node

Internodal atrial conduction pathways

AV node

Bundle of His

Left bundle branch

Right bundle branch

Purkinje fibers

Fig. 2.2 The electrical pathway of the heart starts at the SA node, travels out and across the atria and collects at the AV node. From there, the electricity flows over the bundle of His, down the interventricular septum (through the right and left bundle branches) to the ventricular apex through the very fine network of Purkinje fibers, where the electrical impulse dissipates.

not as quickly as the electrical cells) to contract. Since the heart does not contract as one unit, but rather relies on an atrial contraction, a rest, and a subsequent ventricular contraction and rest, the electricity has to flow in such a way that it causes the contractions to occur at the correct times.

Therefore, the electricity travels rapidly from the SA node down through the atria (this takes about 0.003 s) but then can navigate its way through the AV node only relatively slowly (0.06–0.12 s). This delay gives the atria time to contract and relax before the ventricles contract. Once the electricity reaches the bundle of His at the top of the His–Purkinje system that feeds the ventricles, the electricity travels more rapidly again (0.03–0.05 s). By the time the electricity reaches the end of the Purkinje fibers throughout the ventricular myocardium, the electrical energy has dissipated.

Cellular depolarization and repolarization

All cardiac cells are covered with a semi-permeable membrane that allows certain charged particles (ions) to flow in and out of them. The electricity generated by the SA node and traveling through the healthy heart is mainly the result of positively charged sodium and potassium ions that flow through the semi-permeable membrane of the cardiac cell and change its electrical balance.

The concentration of ions in the cardiac cells gives it an electrical potential (sometimes called "membrane potential") which can be measured in voltage (millivolts mV, thousandths of a volt).

In a resting state, a cardiac cell contains a concentration of negative ions within the cell with a large concentration of positive ions surrounding the cell on the outside. The negatives on the inside (anions) and the positives on the outside (cations) line up almost as opposites, and it is from this that the cellular state gets its name as "polarized." There are two poles: the negatives inside the cell and the positives outside the cell. In this polarized state, the cardiac cell still has a measurable electrical potential, known as "resting membrane potential." Resting membrane potential is higher in myocardial cells and lower in the highly specialized cells of the SA node and AV node.

When an electrical impulse reaches a cardiac cell, it causes that cardiac cell to become permeable to positively charged sodium ions. Positive ions start to flow into the cell, shifting the balance inside the cell from negative to less negative. This decreases the cell's resting membrane potential. When the cell's resting membrane potential falls below a certain level, fast sodium channels open. Just like they sound, fast sodium channels are pores in the cell membrane that allow a quick inflow of positively charged sodium ions. The result is that the inside of the cell quickly becomes positively charged while the cells clustered around the outside are now more negative than positive. Basically, the cell's polarized state is now reversed – or depolarized. The cell's inside is positive and the exterior is mostly negative.

Depolarization causes the myocardial cells to contract, and when they do, positively charged sodium ions start to escape from the interior of the cardiac cell. This outflow of positive ions returns the cardiac cell to its polarized state: negative on the inside with mostly positive ions on the outside. This is known as repolarization or the relaxing of the heart muscle cells as they resume their old shape.

Repolarization is actually a much more complex cellular process than described, involving sodium, calcium and potassium ions. For the purposes of understanding cardiac conduction, these details are not as important as understanding that depolarization and repolarization are cellular processes involving the flow of ions across a cardiac cell membrane.

Fast sodium channels are present in most cardiac electrical cells; these allow the cells to depolarize quickly. The highly specialized cells of the SA node and the AV node do not have fast sodium channels, which would allow them to conduct electricity too quickly. Instead, they have slow calcium-sodium channels. These channels also permit positive ions to enter the cell membrane, but at a much slower rate than the fast sodium channels. The result is that the SA node and the AV node depolarize at significantly slower rates than the rest of the cells in the conduction system.

The action potential

The best way to illustrate the process of depolarization and repolarization of a cardiac cell is through a diagram showing the five phases of polarization (they are numbered zero through four) (Fig. 2.3).

- **Phase 0** is also known as the depolarization phase. An electrical impulse has arrived at a cardiac cell and caused positively charged sodium ions to flow into the cell's interior. This causes the membrane potential to reach what is known as "threshold potential" or the trigger point at which the fast sodium channels open. The fast sodium channels allow a sudden influx of positive sodium ions into the cell. The interior of the cell is now positively charged (instead of negatively charged, as it was at rest). In fact, it is probably about 20 mV more positive than its exterior. Myocardial cells contract.
- **Phase 1** is called the "early rapid repolarization phase." The fast sodium channels close, halting the flow of positive ions into the cell. Meanwhile, positively charged potassium ions flow out of the cell. This decreases the positive charge within the cell to about 0 mV.
- **Phase 2** is the "plateau phase" in which some complex chemical transfers across the cell membrane take place, all while the resting membrane potential remains at around 0 mV. Slow calcium channels in the cardiac cells open, allowing calcium to enter as potassium continues to exit. During this time, the myocardial cells continue the relatively slow process of repolarizing or relaxing.
- **Phase 3** is the "terminal phase of rapid repolarization," characterized by the cardiac cell returning to

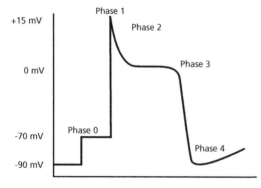

Fig. 2.3 The action potential involves five phases, numbered 0 through 4. The heart begins and ends at its stable resting membrane potential value of about –90 mV. At the point of ventricular depolarization (phase 0) membrane potential changes from negative to positive, then plateaus at around 0 mV before resuming resting membrane potential in phase 4.

its resting membrane potential of about –90 mV. On the cellular level, potassium continues to flow out of the cell membrane and the interior of the cell returns to a negative state while the exterior area surrounding the cell is primarily positive. The myocardial cells are now finished repolarizing or relaxing.
- **Phase 4** could be called "the period between action potentials." While the resting membrane potential has returned to its original resting value of around –90 mV, the cardiac cell still does not have the proper balance of sodium and potassium. There is too much sodium inside the cell and too much potassium outside the cell. At this point, the cell membrane becomes temporarily impermeable to sodium and a mechanism called the "sodium-potassium pump" is initiated. This mechanism pumps sodium out and allows potassium (but not sodium) back into the cell. This complex system is the reason that cardiac cells have a stable resting membrane potential between polarizations.

How polarizations make the heart contract

Whenever one cardiac cell depolarizes (or shifts in electrical balance), it causes adjacent cardiac cells to depolarize. Thus, the heart beats by depolarizing cells, one at a time, starting from the top and moving to the bottom. After depolarization, the cells relax or repolarize. This creates a pattern of electrical energy that can be picked up from the body's skin surface and recorded in a series of waveforms known as the electrocardiogram (ECG or EKG).

The orderly contraction and effective pumping function of the heart depend on the ability of the cells to respond in the proper sequence to electrical stimulation. For this reason, cardiac cells have refractory periods or periods of time during which they cannot be stimulated to depolarize. Put another way, this means cardiac cells are only able to depolarize at certain very specific times.

The refractory period of cardiac cells has two phases. The first is the absolute refractory period (ARP) during which cells are not repolarized, so depolarization is absolutely impossible. The second is the relative refractory period (RRP) during which it takes a powerful jolt of electrical energy to depolarize the heart.

Mapping these refractory periods onto the action potential phases, the absolute refractory period lasts from phase 0 to halfway through phase 3. The relative refractory period occurs in the latter half of phase 3. As the cardiac cells emerge from phase 3, there is a very brief period called the "supernormal period," during which the cell is particularly vulnerable to depolarization. In fact, even a weak electrical stimulus can depolarize the heart during this short phase. After the "supernormal period," the cells enter phase 4 and are susceptible to depolarization at normal electrical energy. All cardiac cells are "excitable" in that they have the ability to polarize or depolarize in response to an electrical stimulus during the fourth phase of the action potential (Fig. 2.4).

Automaticity

The heart is unique in the body in that it possesses the property of automaticity, the ability to automatically generate an electrical output. Automatic-ity is the common characteristic of the specialized cells in the sinoatrial (SA) node located in the high right atrium. A healthy SA node can automatically depolarize itself at the right moment and allow this depolarization wave to travel through the heart's electrical conduction system.

The rate of spontaneous depolarization depends on the slope of phase 4 depolarization of the cardiac cell. A healthy SA node has electrical cells which have a very steep phase 4 upward slope. The steeper the slope, the faster the rate of impulse formation. Cardiac cells with flatter phase 4 slopes depolarize much more slowly (Fig. 2.5).

Increase in sympathetic activity or the presence of catecholamines have the ability to make the phase 4 depolarization slope steeper, that is, to allow the electrical cells of the heart to automatically generate an electrical impulse faster. Parasympathetic activity and certain drugs (lidocaine, procainamide,

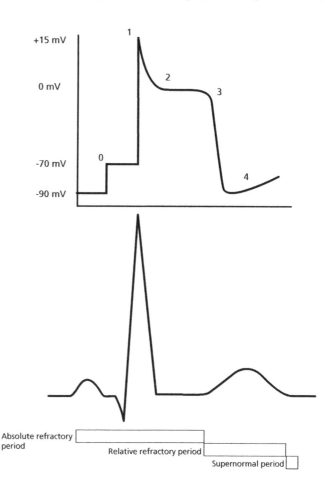

Fig. 2.4 The action potential describes at a cellular level what is going on in the ECG. The ventricular depolarization (the large spike) corresponds to the sudden shift of membrane potential from negative to positive. The T wave corresponds to the point during which the heart cells resume their normal resting potential.

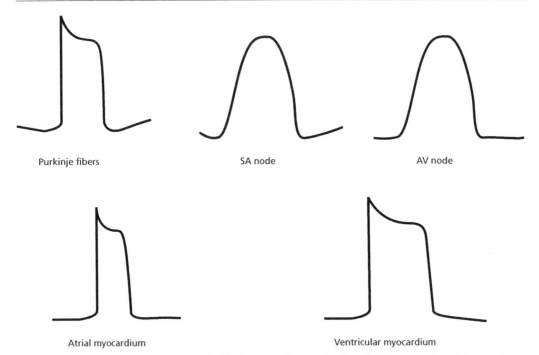

Purkinje fibers   SA node   AV node

Atrial myocardium   Ventricular myocardium

Fig. 2.5 While the overall membrane potential of the heart was illustrated in Fig. 2.4, different portions of the heart's specialized cells actually have slightly different shaped membrane potentials.

quinidine, among others) can flatten the phase 4 depolarization slope and thus decrease the automaticity of these cells. This is how these types of drugs work to increase heart rate (sympathetic activity, catecholamines increase heart rate) or decrease heart rate (parasympathetic activity and drugs like lidocaine, procainamide, and quinidine, among others, slow the heart down).

The SA node is not the only part of the heart that can automatically generate an electrical impulse. In fact, many parts of the heart, including the AV node and the His–Purkinje network, are all capable of firing an electrical impulse. In a healthy heart, the SA node has the most rapid rate of generating electrical impulses.

Once the SA node and its pacemaker cells fire, the other more slowly responding cells get shut out in a process called "overdrive suppression." Basically, this means that the electrical pathway of the heart can only accommodate one impulse at a time, and the first impulse wins. Slower impulses might occur, but they travel to cells during their refractory periods when they cannot respond to depolarization. As a result, the SA node is the dominant pacemaker of the healthy heart. If the SA node becomes diseased

or injured, another portion of the heart may take over to generate electrical impulses. These so-called "escape pacemakers" typically cause the heart to beat at a rate much slower than would be driven by a healthy SA node.

Disorders of the conduction system

The healthy conduction system allows a depolarization, initiated at the proper moment by the SA node, to travel throughout the heart and cause it to beat and relax. The conduction system is the "electrical system" that drives the pumping action of the pump. Many things can adversely impact the heart's electrical system. Conduction disorders can occur in a heart that is otherwise healthy, but conduction disorders also occur frequently with other forms of heart disease.

The two main types of conduction disorders can be described as bradycardia (in which the heart beats too slowly) and tachycardia (in which the heart beats too quickly). Bradycardia can cause mild to profound symptoms of fatigue, dizziness, fainting, and malaise. Tachycardia is typically symptomatic (palpitations, racing heart, pounding in the chest, dizziness, loss of consciousness) and in the extreme form (ventricular fibrillation) may be fatal.

Conduction disorders fall into three main categories. First, there are SA node disorders in which the SA node fails to generate electrical impulses properly. This typically leads to bradycardia, as a much slower escape rhythm takes over.

Second, there are various degrees of heart block in which the electrical pathway of the heart gets slowed or even blocked completely at the AV node. In these cases, the SA node may fire correctly, but the electrical signal gets scrambled, delayed, or even ignored at the AV node. This also produces bradycardia because the ventricles no longer respond to the SA node, but must be driven by a slower escape rhythm. In addition, heart block can create other symptoms as the atrial activity and the ventricular activity become increasingly disorganized. The heart no longer pumps efficiently and the person with heart block can feel easily tired, out of breath, dizzy, and uncomfortable.

The third main type of rhythm disorder is caused by a reentry circuit in the heart's conduction pathways. In a healthy heart, the electrical pathway starts at the top and works its way down to the apex of the ventricles, by which time the energy has dissipated. A reentry circuit forms an endless loop that allows one electrical impulse to travel to and stimulate the same cardiac cells over and over and over again. Instead of progressing through the heart and dissipating, this reentry circuit allows one signal to cause the heart to keep beating faster and faster, even as the SA node continues to generate more electrical signals. This creates tachycardia or too-rapid beating of the heart.

Tachycardia is generally described by the location where the rhythm disorder originates: atrial tachycardia refers to too-rapid beating that originates in the upper chambers, while ventricular tachycardia refers to an excessively high rate originating in the ventricles. Although atrial tachycardia refers to a rapid heart rate that originates in the atria (and one that affects the atria), it can also have ventricular consequences. A supraventricular tachycardia is any tachycardia whose origin is above the ventricles (the atria or the AV node).

Rhythm disorders may be occasional, intermittent, or permanent. While one type of rhythm disorder frequently dominates, it is not unusual for a person to have multiple rhythm disorders. And the problem can get even more complicated in that rhythm disorders may occur suddenly, with or without symptoms.

The main types of cardiac rhythm disorders discussed in this book are described briefly in Table 2.1. These definitions are not meant to be complete and clinical; they are thumbnail sketches.

Further reading

Fogoros RN. *Electrophysiologic Testing: Practical Cardiac Diagnosis Series.* Cambridge, MA: Blackwell Science, 1994.

Huszar RJ. *Basic Dysrhythmias: Interpretation and Management.* St Louis, MO: C. V. Mosby, 1988.

Table 2.1 Types of dysrhythmias

Bradycardia (Fig. 2.6)	*Any rhythm disorder where the heart beats too slowly.*
Sick sinus syndrome (SSS)	Bradycardia caused by the fact that the SA node releases electrical output pulses too slowly, too erratically, or not at all.
Heart block or AV block (AVB)	Any rhythm disorder where the heart beats too slowly or out of synch because the electrical impulse gets blocked (entirely or partially) at the AV node.
First-degree heart block or AVB (Fig. 2.7)	The least severe form of heart block, in which signals get delayed but not blocked in the AV node. It typically appears on an ECG as pauses (sinus arrest), but the relationship of atrial to ventricular activity remains normal (1:1 AV synchrony).
Second-degree heart block or AVB (Figs 2.8 and 2.9)	Heart block in which not all of the impulses from the atria conduct through to the ventricles. This rhythm disorder consists of two types. In Type I (also known as Wenckebach), there is a gradual lengthening of the PR interval until a P wave appears by itself, without a QRS complex. In Type II, the PR interval is stable but a P wave appears intermittently without a corresponding QRS complex, often in a distinct ratio, for example 2:1 block (every second P wave is missing the QRS complex).

Continued p.14

Table 2.1 *Continued.*

Third-degree heart block or AVB or complete heart block (Fig. 2.10)	Heart block in which all impulses are blocked and the atria function independently of the ventricles. Complete heart block may be acquired or congenital.
Tachycardia	Any rhythm disorder where the heart beats too quickly.
Atrial tachycardia	Any rhythm disorder in which the atria beat too quickly. If the atrial impulses conduct through to the ventricles, there can be a rapid ventricular response to the atrial tachycardia, causing a rapid heartbeat. Atrial tachycardia is a collective term for any atrial rate that is too high.
Atrial flutter	A specific type of atrial tachycardia seen on an ECG with a distinctive sawtooth pattern. The atria beat too quickly, usually > 250–350 bpm If the heart has a sound conduction system, this may cause a rapid ventricular response.
Atrial fibrillation (AF) (Fig. 2.11)	A specific type of atrial tachycardia in which the atria beat very rapidly, anywhere above 300 bpm Unlike the much rarer form of atrial flutter, AF is a disorganized rhythm. If the conduction system is intact (or even somewhat functional) there will be a rapid ventricular response. One of the consequences of AF is the dissociation of atrial and ventricular activity. AF is a progressive rhythm disorder.
Paroxysmal AF	AF that comes on suddenly and resolves without intervention. It may occur occasionally or frequently and is frequently asymptomatic.
Persistent AF	AF that comes on suddenly and requires medical intervention (drugs or cardioversion) to convert.
Permanent or chronic AF	AF that occurs all of the time and is refractory to treatment. AF is a progressive disorder that moves gradually from paroxysmal to permanent.
Ventricular tachycardia or VT	Any rhythm disorder caused by a reentry circuit that originates in the ventricles and causes them to beat too quickly. This is a collective term for any type of ventricular rate that is too rapid. VT may or may not respond to drug therapy.
Ventricular fibrillation or VF	The most dangerous dysrhythmia, in which the ventricles beat > 285 times/min. Left untreated, VF is fatal in 4 or 5 min. VF is the cause of "sudden cardiac death" (SCD) also known as "sudden cardiac arrest" (SCA).
Supraventricular tachycardia or SVT	A collective term for any rhythm disorder that originates above the ventricles (in the atria or AV node). This causes too-rapid atrial rates, and if the conduction system is intact, a too-rapid ventricular response.
Brady-tachy syndrome (Fig. 2.12)	An irregular heart rhythm that varies between very slow and fast rates.

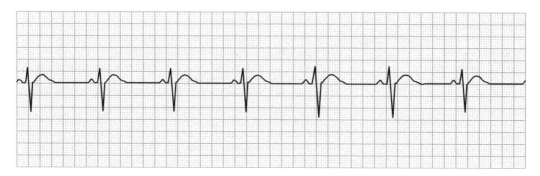

Fig. 2.6 Sinus bradycardia looks like a normal ECG but the rate is much slower, typically < 60 bpm

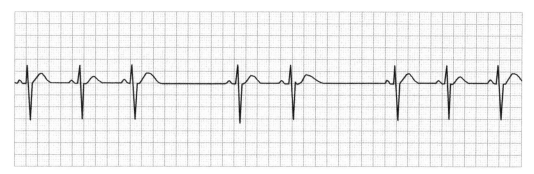

Fig. 2.7 Sinus arrest will cause a pause on the ECG. The length of the pause can vary considerably. People with this rhythm disorder are often asymptomatic, particularly if pauses are short.

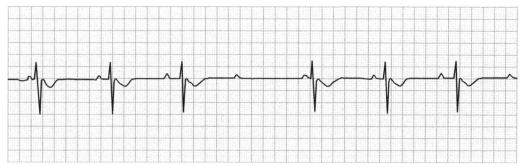

Fig. 2.8 Type I second-degree AV block is also known as Mobitz I or Wenckebach. All of these terms describe a type of rhythm disorder in which not all of the impulses generated by the SA node conduct down through the ventricles. In Type I second-degree AV block, the PR interval gradually lengthens until finally a P wave appears in isolation, without a corresponding QRS complex. After that, a P wave appears followed closely by a QRS complex and the cycle continues.

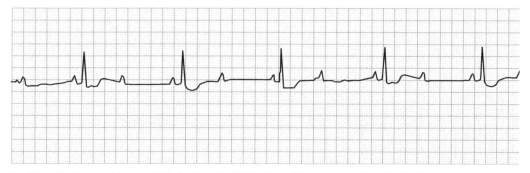

Fig. 2.9 In Type II second-degree AV block, also called Mobitz II, the PR interval remains stable but P waves appear without a corresponding QRS complex. There may be a regular pattern of P waves to QRS complexes expressed as a ratio. For example, 2:1 Mobitz II means there are two P waves for every QRS complex, or, put another way, that every other P wave has no associated QRS complex.

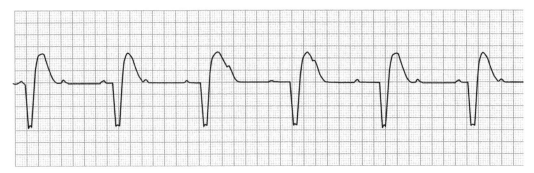

Fig. 2.10 Third-degree AV block is the most severe form of heart block, in which no impulses from the atria conduct through to the ventricles. Also known as complete heart block, this condition involves total dissociation of atria and ventricles. It is the only form of heart block in which a pacemaker is indicated, even if the patient has no symptoms.

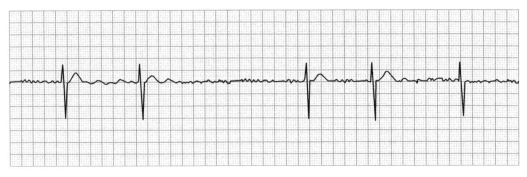

Fig. 2.11 Atrial fibrillation involves disorganized, rapid atrial activity, shown here by the many P waves. In this particular strip, there is only slow and irregular ventricular response to the atrial fibrillation. Sometimes atrial fibrillation can provoke a rapid ventricular response.

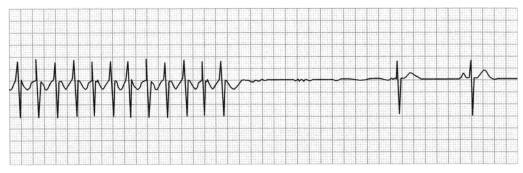

Fig. 2.12 Brady-tachy syndrome is an irregular rhythm that can vary between very slow rates and very rapid rates. It typically involves a supraventricular tachycardia with a rapid response (creating tachycardia portions of the rhythm) and then periods when there is very slow atrial activity or a ventricular escape rhythm.

The nuts and bolts of the conduction system

- The electrical cells in the heart allow for the flow of electricity through a network of gap junctions (electrical cells) that conducts electricity.
- In the healthy heart, the electrical impulse begins in the sinoatrial (SA) node in the high right atrium and conducts downward toward the ventricular apex.
- In the healthy heart, the electrical energy starts from the SA node, proceeds downward toward the atrioventricular (AV) node where it gathers and is delayed slightly before traveling down the ventricles.
- All cardiac cells are covered with a semi-permeable membrane that allows charged particles (ions) to flow in and out of them. The concentration of ions in cardiac cells gives it an electrical potential, sometimes called the membrane potential. Resting membrane potential of the healthy heart is about –90 mV.
- When an electrical impulse reaches a cardiac cell, the cell becomes permeable to positively charged sodium ions. Positive ions flow into the cell, decreasing membrane potential and opening fast sodium channels that cause the interior of the cell to become positively charged. The cell's polarized state is now reversed; it is "depolarized."
- There are five phases of polarization known as phases 0 through 4 of the "action potential." This is a complicated process but basically the cardiac cell changes polarity (from negative to positive and back to negative on the interior) in a way that can be measured in mV.
- Cardiac cells have refractory periods that can be divided into two phases: absolute (when depolarization is impossible) and relative (which means depolarization can occur but only with a large electrical stimulus).
- The heart is unique in the body in that it possesses automaticity, meaning it can automatically generate electricity. Automaticity is a property of the SA node of the heart.
- There are two main categories of conduction disorders: bradycardia (heart beats too slowly) and tachycardia (heart beats too quickly).
- There are three main mechanisms for conduction disorders: disorders of the SA node, heart block (disorders of the AV node), and reentry tachycardias.
- Tachycardias are generally described by where the abnormality originates: an atrial tachycardia originates in the atrium. An atrial tachycardia may affect the ventricles, but it is called "atrial" because the mechanism of origin is in the atrium.
- Rhythm disorders may be occasional, intermittent, or chronic. It is not unusual for one person to have more than one type of rhythm disorder.

CHAPTER 3

Indications for pacing

To determine if a patient will benefit from permanent cardiac pacing, the physician has to take many factors into account. Among these factors are symptoms, underlying etiology, drug therapy, comorbidities, age of the patient, and whether or not the conditions for pacing might resolve. New clinical studies as well as technological innovations from pacemaker companies have significantly expanded indications for pacemakers.

Since the decision to implant a pacemaker may depend on weighing a variety of factors, the American College of Cardiology (ACC) and the American Heart Association and the North American Society of Pacing and Electrophysiology (now known as the Heart Rhythm Society) use a class system in their *Guidelines for the Implantation of Cardiac Pacemakers and Antiarrhythmic Devices*. These classes are described in Table 3.1.

The key element in reaching a decision to implant a pacemaker usually involves the presence of a *documented, symptomatic bradycardia*. Symptomatic bradycardia is defined as a bradyarrhythmia (slower-than-normal heart rate) that is directly responsible for the clinical manifestation of any of the following symptoms: syncope, light-headedness, dizziness, confused states resulting from cerebral hypoperfusion, fatigue, exercise intolerance, hypotension, chest discomfort, or heart failure.

It is important to be able to document the connection between the symptom and the bradycardia. This can be accomplished through a Holter monitor, ambulatory testing carried out in the clinic, an ECG, stress tests, or even electrophysiological testing.

A slow heart rate alone (without symptoms) is not enough to indicate pacemaker therapy. Low heart rates can be physiological, as in the case of athletes in peak condition, or age related, as in young adults. Symptoms alone (without a low heart rate) can be caused by a variety of other conditions, probably unrelated to the heart rate.

In the early days of pacing, AV block was the most common conduction disorder for which a pacemaker was prescribed. While indications have expanded considerably, AV block remains one of the main indications for permanent pacing. Pacing for AV block remains important because even today, no acceptable alternative treatment options exist.

There are several different variations of AV block (and to add to the confusion, some have more than one name) and not all are symptomatic. AV block must be understood as a progressive disorder that delays and ultimately blocks conduction of the electrical impulse through the AV node into the ventricles.

First-degree AV block occurs when the electrical signal produced by the SA node gets delayed

Table 3.1 ACC/AHA/HRS (NASPE) classes

Class	Description
I	Conditions for which there is evidence and/or general agreement that a given procedure or treatment is beneficial, useful, and effective
II	Conditions for which there is conflicting evidence and/or a divergence of opinion about the usefulness/efficacy of a procedure or treatment
IIa	Weight of evidence/opinion is in favor of usefulness/efficacy
IIb	Usefulness/efficacy is less well established by evidence/opinion
III	Condition for which there is evidence and/or general agreement that a procedure/treatment is not useful/effective and in some cases may be harmful

The Nuts and Bolts of Cardiac Pacing, 2nd edition. By Tom Kenny. © 2008 St Jude Medical, ISBN: 978-1-4501-8403-8.

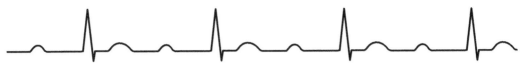

Fig. 3.1 First-degree AV block showing the characteristic long but stable PR interval. Many patients with first-degree AV block are asymptomatic, and, for them, no pacing is indicated. Some patients with asymptomatic first-degree AV block and a long PR interval (> 40 ms) with compromised left-ventricular function may be indicated for an implantable cardioverter-defibrillator.

slightly at the AV node before it can make its way to the ventricles. This manifests on a surface ECG as an abnormally long PR interval, typically defined as a PR segment that lasts 200 ms or longer (Fig. 3.1). First-degree AV block is considered the most benign form of AV block. In fact, many patients are asymptomatic and, for them, no treatment may be the recommended course of action. If first-degree AV block is asymptomatic, it is a Class III indication (no pacing indicated). Even if documented symptoms are present, first-degree heart block is rated as a Class IIa indication.

Second-degree AV block may seem at first glance to be the most complicated form of rhythm disorder, if only for the nomenclature. There are two types of second-degree AV block, known as Type I (also called Mobitz I) and Type II (Mobitz II), named for Woldemar Mobitz, a Russian-born surgeon who worked in Germany in the first half of the 20th century. To further complicate the naming of various forms of second-degree AV block, Type I or Mobitz I second-degree AV block is also called Wenckebach behavior, after another physician who described it. Karel Frederik Wenckebach was a German physician who wrote extensively on rhythm disorders in the early 20th century. Some physicians

write about Type I second-degree AV block as Mobitz Type I. Further compounding the name issue is the fact that names are sometimes used inconsistently; for instance, Type I second-degree AV block may be called Wenckebach by the same author who refers to Type II second-degree AV block as Mobitz II (see Table 3.2).

Type I second-degree AV block is characterized by a progressive prolongation of the PR interval before a blocked beat; usually, the QRS complex is narrow (Fig. 3.2). It differs from first-degree AV block in that first-degree AV block exhibits a stable, but prolonged PR duration. In Type I second-degree AV block, as the PR interval gets longer, the RP interval gets shorter. The RP will eventually shorten to the point that a P wave falls into the refractory period and is blocked.

Table 3.2 Names for second-degree AV block

This condition is the same as:		
Second-degree AV block Type I	Mobitz I	Wenckebach
Second-degree AV block Type II	Mobitz II	

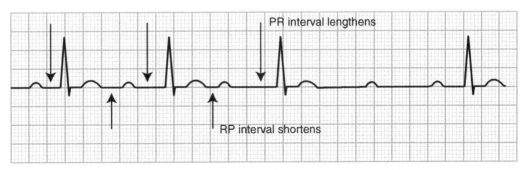

Fig. 3.2 Type I second-degree AV block exhibits a progressively lengthening PR segment until finally a P wave appears on the rhythm strip without an associated QRS complex.

Type II second-degree AV block may take on a couple of classic forms on a rhythm strip, but all of them involve two things: a stable PR interval and a periodic missing QRS complex (i.e. there is a P wave but no associated QRS complex) (Fig. 3.3). The QRS complex may be wide, or at least wider than is common in Type I second-degree AV block. The missing QRS complex may appear intermittently or it may appear in a regular sequence, described in a ratio. For example, 2:1 Type II second-degree AV block means there are two P waves for every one QRS complex (Fig. 3.4). The most frequently encountered ratios for Type II second-degree AV block of this sort are 2:1 and 3:1.

Any form of second-degree AV block, i.e. Type I or Type II, is a Class I pacing indication if accompanied by documented symptoms. Asymptomatic Type I AV block is a Class III indication (i.e. pacing is not indicated) if the block is located at supra-His level, that is, in the AV node (Fig. 3.5). If the block in asymptomatic Type I AV block is located at the intra-His or infra-His levels, it is considered a Class IIa indication, meaning pacing might be beneficial. If documented symptoms are present, any second-degree AV block is an indication for pacing (Class I).

Third-degree AV block defines the absence of AV conduction; impulses originate from the SA node but do not travel through the AV node into the ventricles (Fig. 3.6). As a result, the ventricles beat at the junctional or escape rhythm, independently from atrial activity. Third-degree AV block, sometimes called complete heart block, can be pathological but may also be caused by surgical ablation of the AV junction or certain neuromuscular diseases (such as myotonic muscular dystrophy and others). It may also be congenital. Third-degree AV block with symptoms is a Class I pacing indication, in that expert consensus believes pacing is beneficial for such patients. Many experts recommend a pacemaker for any patient with third-degree AV block, even in the absence of symptoms. In fact, according to the *Guidelines*, this is the only rhythm disturbance (at rates < 40 bpm) that does not require symptoms for indication of a pacemaker. A guide to the various degrees of AV block is given in Table 3.3.

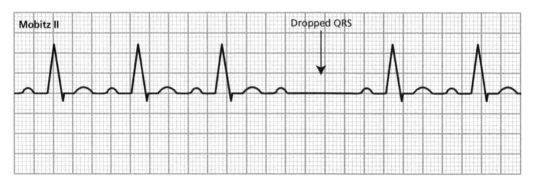

Fig. 3.3 A dropped QRS complex characterizes Type II second-degree AV block. The PR intervals are stable and consistent, and the QRS is wide.

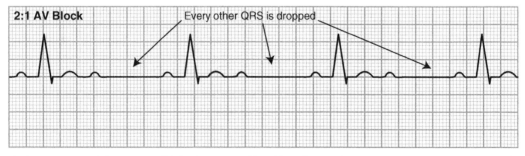

Fig. 3.4 Type II second-degree 2:1 AV block. The PR interval is stable and every other QRS complex is dropped. This type of rhythm disorder might also be called 2:1 AV block.

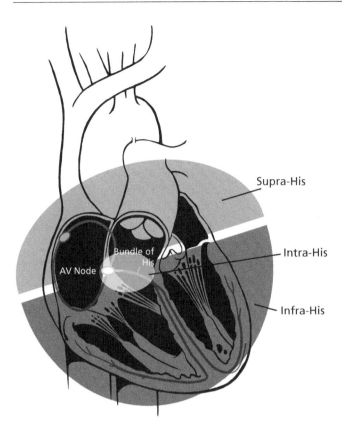

Fig. 3.5 Asymptomatic second-degree Type I AV block is not an indication for pacing if the block occurs at the supra-His level, but pacing may be beneficial (Class IIa) if the block is at the intra-His or infra-His level.

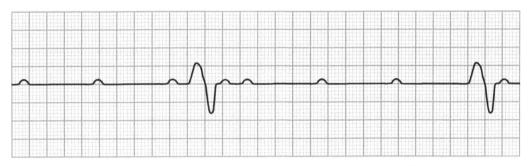

Fig. 3.6 Third-degree AV block occurs when no signals from the atria conduct to the ventricles. The result is complete dissociation of atrial and ventricular activity. This is the most severe form of AV block and pacemakers are a Class IIa indication, even when the patient has no symptoms.

Patients with syncope may have a problem in their bundle branch system. When examined closely, the left bundle branch is found to have two distinct branches: the left anterior and a left posterior fascicle. Conduction system disease can affect one or both branches. When both branches are affected, the result is called left bundle branch block (LBBB) (Fig. 3.7). However, if only one fascicle is affected, the result is called fascicular block.

Development of a block of one fascicle in a patient is called either a left anterior or a left posterior hemiblock. However, if this hemiblock occurs in the setting of right bundle branch block (RBBB), the patient now has bifascicular block.

A patient who has suffered an acute myocardial infarction (MI) may require temporary pacing, but this is not by itself a reason to assume that the patient will have a permanent pacing indication.

Table 3.3 A fast guide to the various degrees of AV block

Name	PR duration	QRS complex	Characteristics	Also known as
First-degree AV block	Longer than 200 ms but stable	Often narrow, "normal"	Stable but prolonged PR segment	
Type I second-degree AV block	Progressively lengthening PR interval and occasional missed QRS complex	May be wide	An occasional missed QRS complex and stable pattern of progressively lengthening PR intervals	Type I Mobitz I Wenckebach
Type II second-degree AV block	Progressively lengthening PR interval and missing QRS complex in a regular pattern, often described as 2:1 or 3:1	May be wide	Steady pattern of missing QRS complexes in a 2:1 or 3:1 ratio (most typical)	Type II Mobitz II
Third-degree AV block	Irregular	May be wide	Complete dissociation of atrial and ventricular activity	Complete heart block

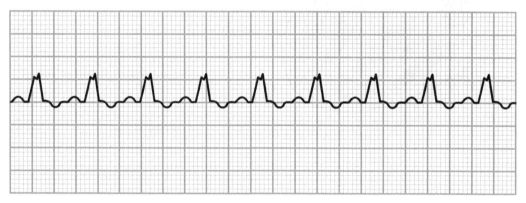

Fig. 3.7 Left bundle branch block (LBBB) with its characteristic notch in the QRS complex. When any bifascicular block occurs with some form of second-degree AV block, pacing is indicated.

Patients with AV block and a prior MI may be indicated for permanent pacing. Unlike other pacing indications, pacing for patients with AV block and a past MI does not depend on symptoms. For heart attack survivors, persistent first-degree AV block does not warrant pacing (Class III), but persistent second-degree AV block – even without symptoms – does (Class I). Generally, the decision to implant a permanent pacemaker in heart attack survivors with some form of AV block is not straightforward and may require considerable analysis. Pacemakers should not be implanted if the peri-infarctional AV block is expected to resolve.

Sinus node dysfunction is the most common arrhythmic constellation that indicates pacing. Sinus node dysfunction is a global term – also called sick sinus syndrome or SSS – that describes sinus bradycardia, sinus arrest, sinoatrial (SA) block, and paroxysmal supraventricular tachyarrhythmias which alternate with bradycardic spells and even asystole. Sinus bradycardia often looks like a normal ECG tracing, except that the rate is insufficient to support the patient (Fig. 3.8). Sinus arrest creates pauses on the ECG, which may or may not prompt symptoms in the patient; the length and frequency of the pauses is decisive. Sinus node dysfunction may manifest itself as chronotropic incompetence, i.e. an inadequate cardiac response to meet the body's needs during times of exercise or stress. Any type of sinus node dysfunction with associated, documented symptoms is a Class I pacing indication.

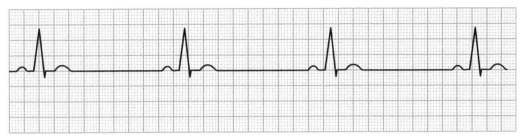

Fig. 3.8 Sinus bradycardia which appears like a "normal" ECG but at a slower rate. If the patient has symptoms, this is a Class I pacing indication.

In some cases, pacemakers can help prevent certain arrhythmias. Continuous pacing has been shown to prevent ventricular tachycardia in some patients with congenital long-QT syndrome (drug therapy may also be recommended along with pacing). Patients with tachyarrhythmias induced by pauses may benefit from cardiac pacing, which eliminates the pauses that trigger the arrhythmias. In fact, pacemakers often benefit patients with brady-tachy syndrome, a rhythm disorder characterized by periods of too-rapid and too-slow heart rates (Fig. 3.9). The advantage of pacing in brady-tachy syndrome is that it allows the physician to give the patient drugs to treat the tachycardic phase of the syndrome without worrying about worsening the bradycardia.

Hypersensitive carotid sinus syndrome, an extreme reflex response to carotid sinus stimulation, can cause syncope or presyncope in susceptible patients. Hyperactive response is defined as response to carotid massage which provokes one or both of:
- asystole of 3 s or more owing to either sinus arrest or AV block
- a substantial symptomatic decrease in systolic blood pressure.

Since pauses of up to 3 s during carotid sinus massage are not considered abnormal, the diagnosis of hypersensitive carotid sinus syndrome must be made carefully. If a patient complains of syncope that can be reproduced by carotid sinus massage, it indicates hypersensitive response.

To evaluate whether a person with hypersensitive carotid sinus syndrome is a candidate for pacing, the clinician needs to evaluate the two components of the condition (Table 3.4). First, there is a cardioinhibitory response, which results from increased parasympathetic tone. This manifests as any or all of the following: decreased sinus rate, prolonged PR interval, or advanced AV block. Second, there is a vasodepressor response, caused by reduced sympathetic activity and resulting in loss of vascular tone and hypotension. The vasodepressor response is independent of changes in heart rate.

The majority of patients with hypersensitive carotid response have a significant cardioinhibitory response component and are considered candidates for pacing (Class I) if they have recurrent syncope or ventricular systole longer than 3 s caused by carotid sinus massage. Yet a hypersensitive carotid response

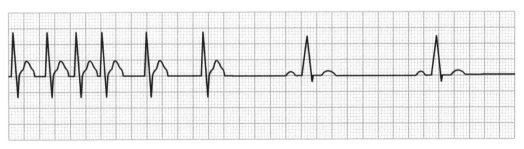

Fig. 3.9 Brady-tachy syndrome consists of periods of tachycardia (too-rapid heart rate) and bradycardia (too-slow heart rate). The tachycardia is triggered by pauses in the heart rhythm. A pacemaker eliminates the pauses, and paces the heart at an appropriate rate.

Table 3.4 Components of hypersensitive carotid sinus syndrome

Component	Results from	Classic symptoms
Cardioinhibitory response	Increased parasympathetic tone	Low sinus rate, prolonged PR interval, advanced AV block
Vasodepressor response	Reduced sympathetic activity	Loss of vascular tone, hypotension

that does not provoke specific symptoms is considered a Class III indication.

Syncope can be one of the most confounding symptoms for cardiologists, since symptoms can trace to a number of different causes (Table 3.5). Neurocardiogenic syncope is a name given to several conditions in which a neural reflex triggers systemic hypotension, characterized by both bradycardia and peripheral vasodilation. A common type of neurocardiogenic syncope is vasovagal syncope, which may involve symptoms of nausea and light sensitivity. Vasovagal syncope can be triggered by pain, stress, anxiety, or crowded conditions and there is evidence to suggest that it may be hereditary. The ACC estimates that from 10% to 40% of all syncopal episodes are neurocardiogenic in origin.

Accompanied by severe symptoms and documented with either spontaneous bradycardic episodes or bradycardia inducible with tilt-table testing, neurocardiogenic syncope is a Class IIa pacing indication (pacing may be useful). Permanent pacing for patients with refractory neurocardiogenic syncope and profound bradycardia or asystole remains controversial, as it often occurs in patients who have no evidence of structural heart disease. But neurocardiogenic syncope does not necessarily mean that the patient has bradycardia; about one-tenth to one-fifth of all neurocardiogenic syncope patients have a predominant vasodepressor

reaction without a significant bradycardia. For such patients with a significant cardioinhibitory component to the neurocardiogenic syncope, at least one study showed that pacing significantly increased the time to the first syncopal event. Although much still remains to be learned about pacing for neurocardiogenic syncope, it seems that the best mode for such patients is DDD (see Chapter 5) with a special rate-drop response feature. In this context, it is important to keep in mind that even when cardiac pacing is indicated for cardioinhibitory syncope, it does not cure the disease, but rather decreases the symptoms of decreased cardiac output.

Other causes for syncope include left ventricular outflow tract obstruction, bradyarrhythmias, and tachycardia. The presence of syncope does not, in and of itself, indicate that a permanent pacemaker is warranted.

In terms of pacemaker indications, the conditions of dilated cardiomyopathy (DCM) and hypertrophic obstructive cardiomyopathy (HOCM) are under considerable scrutiny right now. The presence of either form of cardiomyopathy is not a contraindication to pacing. In fact, cardiomyopathy patients who are otherwise indicated for permanent pacing (for instance, because of sick sinus syndrome or AV block) are considered to have Class I indications for pacemakers. On the other hand, cardiomyopathy patients who have no symptoms or can

Table 3.5 Neurocardiogenic and vasovagal syncope notes

Type	Triggered by	Symptoms	Percentage	When is it a pacing indication?
Neurocardiogenic	Neural reflex	Systemic hypotension, peripheral vasodilation, sometimes bradycardia	10–40% of all syncopal episodes may be neurocardiogenic in origin	Severe symptoms plus documented bradycardia (spontaneous or tilt-table) is Class IIa.
Vasovagal	Vasodepressor reaction	The above plus nausea, light sensitivity	About 25% of neurocardiogenic episodes may be vasovagal	Not all patients will have bradycardia

be effectively managed on drug therapy are contra-indicated for pacing (Class III). This is an area of considerable investigation at the moment.

An emerging indication for cardiac pacemakers is the relatively new population of patients who have received a heart transplant. As many as a quarter of cardiac transplant patients experience bradycardia and these bradyarrhythmias are frequently associated with sinus node dysfunction. Long-term pacing may not be necessary, in that bradycardia resolves in about half of heart transplant patients within the first year. Right now, guidelines indicate permanent pacemakers for transplant patients whose brady-cardia is not expected to resolve and who manifest Class I indications (documented symptomatic bra-dycardia). Transplant patients with asymptomatic bradycardia are contraindicated for pacing (Class III).

Further reading

ACC/AHA/NASPE. *Guidelines Update for Implantation of Cardiac Pacemakers and Antiarrhythmic Devices*, 2002. Accessed from www.naspe.org on 20 November 2004.

Dorostkar PC, Eldar M, Belhassen B *et al.* Long-term follow-up of patients with long-QR syndrome treated with beta-blockers and continuous pacing. *Circulation* 1999; **100**: 2431–6.

Gregoratos G, Cheitlin MD, Conill A *et al.* ACC/AHA Guidelines for implantation of cardiac pacemakers and an-tiarrhythmic devices: executive summary. *Circulation* 1998; **97**: 1325–35.

Oakley, D. *The Athlete's Heart. Heart Online.* Accessed from http://heart.bmjjournals.com on 20 November 2004.

The nuts and bolts about indications for pacing

- The classes established by leading heart specialty societies range from Class I (general agreement that pacing is useful) to Class III (general agreement that pacing would not be useful) with Class II dealing with cases where there is a divergence of clinical opinion. Class IIa occurs when there are differing opinions, but there is evidence that pacing would be useful, while Class IIb occurs when there are differing opinions but the evidence supporting pacing is not that well established.
- The key element in a pacing indication is a documented and symptomatic episode of bradycardia. Bradycardias can be documented through Holter monitoring, ambulatory testing, ECG taken at the clinic, or even electrophysiological studies.
- AV block occurs when the electrical signal gets delayed or even interrupted at the AV node. There are three degrees of AV block, with first degree the least severe and third degree the most severe.
- First-degree AV block has a stable but abnormally prolonged PR interval on the ECG. This is a Class III indication if no symptoms occur; even with symptoms, it is a Class IIa.
- Second-degree AV block may occur as Type I (sometimes called Mobitz I or Wenckebach) or as Type II (sometimes called Mobitz II). Both forms involve dropped QRS complexes.
- In Type I second-degree AV block, the PR interval gets increasingly prolonged until an atrial event does not conduct to the ventricle at all. The QRS is narrow.
- In Type II AV block, QRS complexes get dropped (i.e. an atrial beat occurs without a corresponding ventricular beat) in a 2:1 or 3:1 or other regular pattern.
- Any form of second-degree AV block (Type I or Type II) is a Class I pacing indication if the patient has symptoms.
- Third-degree AV block (sometimes called "complete heart block") occurs when no impulses from the SA node travel through to the ventricles; the atria and ventricles are completely dissociated. This is a Class I indication if the patient has symptoms and is a Class IIa indication, even if the patient is asymptomatic.
- Bundle branch block may occur on the right or left side and is a form of intraventricular conduction disorder. It is evident on an ECG with a characteristic notch in the QRS complex. Persistent second-degree AV block with bilateral bundle branch block is a Class I pacing

Continued p.26

Continued.

indication.
• Sinus node dysfunction is a global term that includes many disorders including sick sinus syndrome, sinus arrest, sinoatrial block or supraventricular tachyarrhythmias. Sinus node dysfunction can also manifest as chronotropic incompetence. Sinus node dysfunction is a Class I pacing indication if the patient has symptoms.
• Hypersensitive carotid response patients may be candidates for pacing if they have recurrent syncope or ventricular systole longer than 3 s provoked by carotid sinus massage. If they do not have symptoms, they are considered to have a Class III (i.e. no) indication for pacing.
• Syncope is, in and of itself, not necessarily an indication for pacing, although it may be caused by any number of conditions that can be treated by a pacemaker. Neurocardiogenic syncope is a subset of syncopal conditions which are considered a Class II pacing indication if the patient has symptoms and can be induced to bradycardia during tilt-table testing.

CHAPTER 4

The history of pacing

The history of pacing and electrophysiology really started with Luigi Galvani (1737–1798) who studied what he called "animal electricity." Around the time that Benjamin Franklin was proving that lightning was a form of electricity, Galvani found that fluids from a dissected frog would conduct electricity when placed between two poles. Later, he discovered that when electrical energy was applied to the leg muscles of dissected frogs, it would cause the muscles to contract.

Galvani himself wrote about what might be called the birth of electrophysiology:

> I had dissected and prepared a frog in the usual way and while I was attending to something else I laid it on a table on which stood an electrical machine at some distance from its conductor and separated from it by a considerable space. Now when one of the persons present touched accidentally and lightly the inner crural nerves of the frog with the point of a scalpel, all the muscles of the legs seemed to contract again and again as if they were affected by powerful cramps.

While Galvani at the University of Bologna in Italy was one of the first pioneers of medical electricity, he found no practical applications for his work.

Meanwhile, another Italian academician, Alessandro Giuseppe Anastasio Volta (1745–1827) developed the prototype of the battery. He fashioned a stack of metallic disks and found it could conduct electricity. Known then as the "voltaic pile," it is the model on which modern-day alkaline batteries are made. Volta discovered that electricity could be conducted through non-organic materials. His early work in electricity included developing a crude forerunner of our modern-day capacitor. The unit of electrical measurement, the volt, was named after him.

The third big name in early electrical research is Michael Faraday (1791–1867) who pioneered what he called "electrochemistry." Faraday was interested in electromagnetic induction and his early work was so prolific that he is credited with having named electrodes, electrolytes, and ions.

In Germany, two academicians named C. Ludwig and Augustus D. Waller devised a capillary electrometer. The device used a sensor, magnets, and electricity to create an electrical field. It was attached to a capillary tube filled with liquid. When electricity was applied to the device, the fluid would rise and fall in response to the electrical energy. Ludwig and Waller immediately saw the value in such a device for measuring physiological electricity, such as the electrical activity of the heart. Unfortunately, the device they fashioned was too crude to accomplish the task, but it did establish the foundation for the next inventor.

One of the most famous names in early pacing history is that of Willem Einthoven (1870–1927), who was professor of physiology at the University of Leiden in Holland. Einthoven won the Nobel Prize for Medicine in 1924 for the electrocardiogram or ECG. Einthoven became intrigued by the capillary electrometer of Ludwig and Waller, and found he could stabilize the instrument to get more accurate readings through a variety of measures, including using photosensitive paper to record results more precise than those obtained by a rising and falling fluid level. Einthoven not only invented the prototype for our modern ECG, he also recognized in his own early research that ECG tracings could be indicative of various forms of heart disease.

The first pacemaker was invented not by a doctor in a laboratory, but by an engineer in his kitchen. It started when Arne Larsson (1915–2001) of Sweden contracted debilitating heart disease. Larsson had complete heart block and severe Stokes–Adams attacks in the 1950s. Medications and other therapies offered little help. Larsson's wife, Else-Marie, heard of animal experiments using electricity on cardiac tissue at Karolinska Hospital – one of Europe's leading hospitals and located in nearby Stockholm, Sweden. She went to Karolinska Hospital to persuade thoracic surgeon Dr Ake Senning (1915–2000) and an engineer named Rune Elmqvist (1906–1996) to develop some sort of device to help her husband.

Rune Elmqvist is one of Sweden's greatest inventors with many breakthroughs to his credit. The pacemaker, built in 1958, was about the size of a hockey puck and contained just two transistors. The greatest challenge to the inventor was the power source. The original pacemaker contained large nickel cadmium cells to power the device.

The first pacemaker was implanted 8 October 1958, in Arne Larsson. The device lasted just 3 h before it stopped working. The first pacemaker revision surgery occurred on 9 October 1958 when Larsson got his second device. This one lasted much longer and was the second in what would become 22 devices Larsson would receive over his lifetime. Although Larsson's early pacemakers were large, unreliable, and did nothing more than pace asynchronously, he became a leading advocate for the advancement of pacemaker therapy. Over the years, Larsson's longevity and enthusiasm proved that pacemakers did more than just keep a person alive; they had the potential to improve quality of life.

Larsson's original pacemakers were rechargeable systems. By wearing a shoulder-pad device and connecting with a power source, the nickel-cadmium batteries could be charged up at regular intervals. The first leads required a thoracotomy for implantation. Pacemakers were possible, but not exactly safe, easy, or convenient.

Around the time that Larsson got the Elmqvist pacemaker in Sweden, a cardiac surgeon working in the Twin Cities area of Minnesota was struggling with the harsh realities of open-heart surgery for the repair of ventricular septal defects. Dr C. Walton Lillehei (1918–1999) found that this surgery produced iatrogenic complete AV block that either resolved or had dire and even lethal consequences for the patient. External pacemakers were used for the immediate postoperative period. On Halloween in 1957, a massive power outage in the Twin Cities cut off power to the hospital where Lillehei worked. External pacemakers were no longer powered. One child may have even died

as a result of the loss of electrical power. Dr Lillehei approached a medical entrepreneur about building an implantable pacemaker.

The medical entrepreneur was Earl Bakken (1924–) who had founded a then-fledgling company called Medtronic. Medtronic started in 1949 more or less in Bakken's garage, which was where he built his first pacemaker. Bakken found a suitable diagram for an electric circuit from a *Popular Mechanics* article about electronic metronomes. Wilson Greatbatch (1919–) is credited with designing the prototype together with Dr William Chardach. The first implantable pacemaker in America was implanted by Dr Lillehei in 1960.

From that point, the history of pacing becomes one long string of innovations. In 1964, Barouh Berkovits (1926–) invented the first demand pacemaker, which is a pacemaker that paces only when pacing is required. Dr Doris Escher (1917–) is credited with the first transvenous pacemaker implant in 1958, but it was not until the mid-1960s that transvenous leads came into widespread use. With a transvenous lead, a patient no longer needed open-chest surgery to receive a pacemaker. The introduction of transvenous lead systems was a major boost for pacemakers.

Seymour Furman invented the world's first transvenous lead, fashioned from a stimulating catheter electrode. Probably no other single individual has done as much to advance the field of cardiac pacing as this Bronx-born physician. A prolific author and speaker, Furman was a tireless advocate for pacing technology. He established the first pacemaker clinics in this country, founded the esteemed journal *Pacing and Clinical Electrophysiology* (PACE), and co-established the organization then known as the North American Society of Pacing and Electrophysiology (NASPE) and today called the Heart Rhythm Society. His long list of achievements would include development of the strength–duration curve (for defining pacemaker outputs), transtelephonic monitoring for pacemakers, and the establishment of the US pacemaker registry. Together with his colleague Doris Escher, Seymour Furman authored the very first American book on pacemakers: *The Principles and Techniques of Cardiac Pacing,* published in 1970.

Up until 1970, all implantable pacemakers relied on the nickel-cadmium batteries of the original

Greatbatch device. Wilson Greatbatch introduced the lithium-iodine battery in 1970, which offered longer service life and more stable decay curves. Lithium-iodine batteries are still in use today and it was battery technology that allowed pacemakers to downsize to the dimensions used today (Fig. 4.1).

Most of the subsequent innovations in cardiac pacing have occurred through the work of manufacturers. Dual-chamber pacing was pioneered in the 1970s; rate-responsive pacing came to the fore-

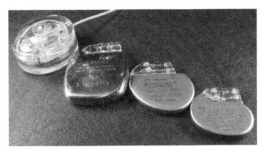

Fig. 4.1 Pacemakers have become smaller and smarter over the years.

front in the 1980s. Lead technology evolved to include screw-in leads (invented by Jacques Mugica, 1933–2002), bidirectional telemetry programmers, extensive programmability, downloadable diagnostics, stored electrograms, mode switching, and other features.

Further reading

Dubin D. *Rapid Interpretation of EKG's*. Tampa, FL: Cover, 1993.

Faraday Biography. Accessed from www.rigb.org on 20 November 2004.

Galvani, L. *De Viribus Electricitatis in Motu Musculari Commentaries*. Bologna: Institute of Science, 1791.

HRS Online. *Notable Figures*. Accessed from www.hrsonline. org/ephistory/notable_figures.

Hurst JW, Conti CR, Fye WB. *Profiles in Cardiology: A Collection of Profiles Featuring Individuals Who Have Made Significant Contributions to the Study of Cardiovascular Disease*. Mahwah, NJ: Clinical Cardiology, 2003.

Lüderiz B. *History of the Disorders of Cardiac Rhythm*. Armonk, NY: Futura, 1995.

Volta Biography. Accessed from www.italian-american.com/ volta.htm on 20 November 2004.

The nuts and bolts of the history of pacing

- The notion of "animal electricity" was known in the 1700s but it was not until electricity could be harnessed in a battery that electrophysiological work could be conducted.
- Modern battery technology derives from the work of an Italian inventor (Alessandro Volta) and an Irish scientist (Michael Faraday).
- Two German scientists, Ludwig and Waller, realized that electricity from the body could be measured, but it took the work of Dutch professor Willem Einthoven to invent the surface ECG in 1924, for which he won the Nobel Prize in Medicine.
- The first pacemaker was invented by a Swedish engineer named Rune Emqvist and implanted in Arne Larsson in 1958. The first pacemaker replacement surgery was performed the next day, when the initially implanted device stopped working. Over his lifetime, Larsson would have

a total of 22 devices; he became an advocate for pacemaker therapy.
- The original pacemakers were rechargeable. It was not until Wilson Greatbatch developed long-lasting battery technology that pacemakers could be self-contained and have long service lives.
- In the United States, Earl Bakken developed an early prototype of the pacemaker based on a diagram for an electric circuit for an electronic metronome that he found in *Popular Mechanics*. Dr C. Walton Lillehei implanted the first pacemaker in America (the Bakken design) in 1960. This prototype is close in concept to what is currently in use today.
- Since the first pacemaker implants, the history of pacing has been a long line of innovation. Transvenous leads made the thoracotomies required in early implants unnecessary. Dual-

Continued p.30

Continued.

chamber systems provided AV synchrony. Bidirectional telemetry and memory allowed clinicians to communicate, change, and download information from implanted pacing systems.

- Battery technology has evolved from nickel-cadmium batteries to today's lithium-iodine batteries. This has allowed pacemakers to downsize while actually increasing in longevity.
- Seymour Furman co-founded NASPE (today HRS), established the *PACE* journal, invented transtelephonic monitoring and transvenous leads, and wrote the first book on cardiac pacing together with Doris Escher. Dr Furman has authored hundreds of books and articles on pacing.

CHAPTER 5

Implantable device codes

Pacemakers were still in their infancy in 1974 when the first pacemaker code was published by a group known as the Intersociety Commission for Heart Disease Resources (ICHD). Clinicians needed a generic, shorthand way of describing pacemakers in terms of functionality. Since that time, the ICHD code has been revised a couple of times – by the North American Society of Pacing and Electrophysiology (NASPE) and the British Pacing Group (BPG) in 1985 and later. A corresponding code for defibrillators was developed in the 1980s. Today, the "official" code for pacemakers and ICDs is known as the NBG code (NBG is a blend of NASPE and BPG) (Table 5.1).

The first letter in the NBG code (called the "first position" in most NBG charts) describes the chamber or chambers that are paced by the device. The NBG code officially allows four possible options, but a fifth one is in widespread unofficial use. Those code letters for the first position are A for atrium, V for ventricle, D for "dual" meaning both atrium and ventricle, and O if no pacing occurs at all. Thus, any pacemaker code that starts with D (DDI, DDDR, DVI, DOO) means that the pacemaker paces in both atrium and ventricle.

Manufacturers building single-chamber pacemakers had difficulty with the A or V designation, since the same single-chamber pacemaker can be used for an atrial as well as a ventricular application. Thus, many companies started using S for single to describe pacemakers that were capable of pacing in one chamber of the physician's choice. Today, S is commonly used and understood, but is not part of the official NBG code. When a physician implants an SSI device into a patient with a lead in the ventricle, the device is more accurately called a VVI pacemaker.

Manufacturers frequently put codes for pacemakers on shipping boxes and in labeling. For such purposes, the generally recognized convention is that the manufacturer states the highest mode the device is capable of pacing. For example, a dual-chamber rate-responsive pacemaker would be properly labeled DDDR, although it could be implanted and programmed to pace DDD or even VVIR.

Mode codes are also used by clinicians to discuss programmable options of devices or functional characteristics of the pacemaker. Such codes can be handy shorthand ways to talk about how the system is programmed or how it is actually functioning in certain situations. For example, a DDD pacemaker with mode switching may sometimes function as a VVI pacemaker when the mode switch algorithm is in effect.

Table 5.1 The NBG code for pacemakers updated in 2000

Position	I	II	III	IV	V
Category	Chamber(s) paced	Chamber(s) sensed	Response to sensing	Rate modulation	Multisite pacing
	O = None	O = None	O = None	O = None	O = None
	A = Atrium	A = Atrium	T = Triggered	R = Rate modulation	A = Atrium
	V = Ventricle	V = Ventricle	I = Inhibited		V = Ventricle
	D = Dual (A+V)	D = Dual (A+V)	D = Dual (T+I)		D = Dual (A+V)
Manufacturer designation only	S = Single (A or V)	S = Single (A or V)			

The second position in the NBG code describes the chamber or chambers in which the device senses or detects signals. The same letters are used: A for atrium, V for ventricle, D for dual or both atrium and ventricle. Manufacturers can use S for "single chamber" and it is understood that this device will only be an A or V device after the physician has chosen the chamber for its application. The letter O may be used to describe a device with no sensing capabilities.

Although the NBG code first came into use to help clinicians describe a variety of new devices, pacemakers for the past few decades are extensively programmable. That programmability extends to modes as well, so the NBG code is sometimes used to describe a programmed mode of a device. As a rule of thumb, the code used to describe a device is the highest or most sophisticated level of programmability in that device. If, for some reason, the device is temporarily or even permanently programmed to a different mode for clinical reasons, the code becomes a handy way to describe the new functionality of the device.

An example of this might be a pacemaker that is labeled in the box as an SSI device. We know from the first two positions that this is a pacemaker that paces and senses in a single chamber only. Once the device is implanted with a ventricular lead and programmed for ventricular application, the device is more correctly described as a VVI pacemaker. If a clinician wanted to do some temporary testing of the device, he might program it to OOO mode (no pacing, no sensing at all) to see the patient's intrinsic rhythm. If he only wants to turn off sensing, he can program the device to VOO. Thus, the NBG code can describe both a device (its highest mode) or a mode of therapy.

The third letter of the NBG code is more complicated in that it describes how the pacemaker responds to a sensed event. If the pacemaker is inhibited, i.e. if it withholds a pacing output pulse in response to a sensed event, then it has an I in the third position. An example of an inhibited device is a VVI device: the pacemaker paces in the ventricle, senses in the ventricle, and when it senses an event in the ventricle, it inhibits or withholds a pacing output. Most single-chamber devices in use are inhibited devices.

If the third letter is T, it means the device responds to a sensed event by triggering or initiating an output pulse. This is the opposite approach of the inhibited device, which does not pace when it senses activity. A triggered device paces into a sensed event. While it is fairly uncommon to see a VVT device in permanent use, many times clinicians will temporarily program triggered modes to evaluate device behavior.

If the third position letter is a D it stands for "dual," meaning the device may be triggered to pace by a sensed event in one chamber and inhibited by a sensed event in the other chamber. A very common mode of operation is DDD: the device paces in both chambers, senses in both chambers, and can respond to sensed activity by inhibiting in one chamber and triggering in the other.

The fourth position in the NBG code adds an R for rate modulation or rate response. A rate-responsive pacemaker varies its rate based on the perceived activity levels of the patient. Thus, an AAIR device paces in the atrium, senses in the atrium, inhibits or withholds a pacing output when it senses atrial activity, and is rate modulated so that the pacing rate increases with activity. For non-rate-modulated devices, it is possible to use an O (no rate modulation) in the fourth position, but common practice often just omits a letter in the fourth position (for example, DDD and DDDR pacemakers).

The R designator in the fourth position applies to any sort of rate modulation: piezoelectric sensor, accelerometer, minute ventilation, even temperature-sensing pacemakers. Thus, R does not tell you what type of rate modulation is in effect, only that the system modulates the rate based on anticipated patient needs using some method. Even pacemakers with advanced dual-sensor technology for rate modulation are identified by code simply with an R.

The fifth position was changed in 2000 to accommodate the need to designate multisite pacing, which means simply pacing at more than one site. An A in this place means that the pacemaker is pacing both right and left atria or is pacing the right atrium in more than one place or both.

A V refers to pacing both both right and left ventricles (so-called "biventricular pacing" or sometimes "cardiac resynchronization therapy") or pacing the right ventricle at two or more sites or both. D indicates either multisite atrial and multisite ventricular pacing, although several variations are possible. For instance, D could be used for a biventricular system that paces the right atrium at two locations. The same D could also refer to a pacemaker equipped to pace right and left ventricles. While any letter other than O (meaning none) in the fifth position indicates some form of multisite pacing, the code does not offer specific details about the form of multisite pacing.

Note that for the purposes of the NBG code, septal pacing to activate both right and left sides of the heart is *not considered* a form of multisite pacing (Fig. 5.1).

While the NBG code can be very practical in describing devices, it by no means can fully express the complexity of rhythm management devices on the market today. New features, extensive programmability, and a variety of timing cycles allow for remarkable fine-tuning of devices. Thus, not all DDDR devices are created equal! But all DDDR devices will pace and sense in both chambers, respond to sensed events by inhibiting in one chamber and triggering in the other, and modulate the pacing rate in response to the patient's needs.

Further reading

Bernstein AD. *Pacemaker, Defibrillator, and Lead Codes*. Accessed from www.hrsonliune.org on 20 November 2004.

Bernstein AD, Daubert J-C, Fletcher RD *et al.* The revised NASPE/BPEG generic code for antibradycardia, adaptive-rate and multisite pacing. *PACE* 2000; **25**: 260–4.

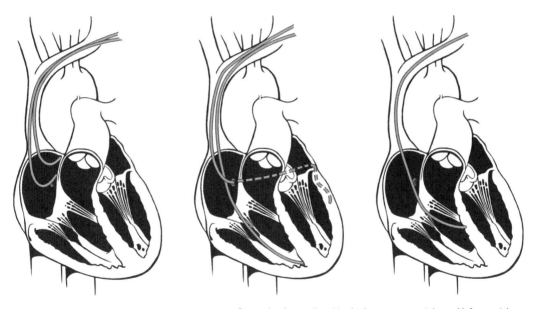

Fig. 5.1 Some new lead locations in cardiac pacing. Left, two leads are placed in the heart to pace right and left ventricles for biventricular pacing, another type of multisite pacing. Right, a ventricular pacing lead is fixated to the ventricular septum to help pace both right and left ventricles together; although this type of pacing stimulates two chambers, it is not considered multisite pacing because there is only one lead location.

The nuts and bolts of the NBG code

- The most commonly used code for pacemakers is the NBG code.
- Devices are labeled by the manufacturer with the highest level code the device is capable of performing. A device labeled DDDR is capable of rate modulation, whether or not the physician decides to turn it on.
- Mode codes are used in product labeling (to show the highest attainable mode the device can achieve) or as a clinical abbreviation for how the device is programmed or is functioning.
- The NBG code requires the use of an A, V, D or O in the first and second position, but many manufacturers label devices with an S (such as an SSIR device). S is taken to mean "single." Such devices can be used for either atrial or ventricular single-chamber application.
- The NBG code was updated in 2000 and the fifth position changed to "multisite pacing." Multisite pacing can occur when both right and left sides of the heart are paced (e.g. both right and left ventricles) or when one chamber is paced at more than one site (for instance, at two sites in the right atrium). As multisite pacing expands and becomes more common, it is possible this designation will increase in significance or change to accommodate device evolution.
- Codes can also be used to designate modes. For example, a physician's manual may suggest temporarily programming a DDD device to VVT for diagnostic purposes.

CHAPTER 6

Pacemaker technology

The pacemaker system consists of four important, interconnected elements:

- the pulse generator or implantable device
- the lead or leads that connect the generator to the heart
- a programmer or patient care system (tabletop computer) that can communicate with the implanted device
- the patient.

As the pulse generator is the "heart" of the system, it is not uncommon to call it the pacemaker, although it requires the interaction of the other three elements to work. The modern pacemaker is not very much like the one that was first implanted decades ago in Arne Larsson – except in theory.

The theory is that a pacemaker should deliver precisely timed, small electrical output pulses. To do this, it requires certain timing mechanisms and a power source for the electricity. As devices became more sophisticated, the tiny mechanisms originally intended to deliver precisely timed outputs also became increasingly sophisticated. Today, it is no exaggeration to consider a pacemaker as a mini-computer (Fig. 6.1). It contains complex circuitry that is capable

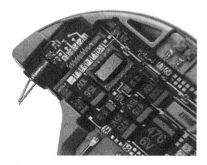

Fig. 6.1 Pacemaker chip technology relies on microelectronics, which allows very intricate electronics in a tiny space. If today's pacing electronics were built using yesterday's transistor technology, then a pacemaker would be too large to implant in a human being.

of analyzing incoming information (from sensing electrodes) and responding appropriately (deciding whether to deliver an output or not, based on what the person's heart is doing). Pacemakers contain memory, and store electrograms from the heart in memory for later download by the clinician during follow-up. While the nuts and bolts of the pacemaker's "brains" are too complex for the scope of this book, there are some important facets that need to be understood about how a pacemaker "thinks."

Pacemakers receive input from the heart through the pacing lead electrodes in a function known as "sensing." The purpose of sensing is to allow the pacemaker to assess what the heart is doing and to pace in response to the patient's intrinsic rhythms (or lack thereof). The input the pacemaker receives comes in the form of electrical energy detected by the lead's electrodes and transferred to the device. The trouble with this method – and one reason that the first pacemakers could not sense at all – is that the human body generates a lot of electrical energy all of the time. Some noises are myopotentials – muscle noise. The electrical energy of the larger ventricles can sometimes drown out the electricity generated by the smaller, weaker atria, to the extent that an atrial lead might pick up ventricular noise. Sorting through all of this energy and arriving at a viable signal from the right chamber posed a major challenge for designers of the earliest pacemakers.

It was solved through a filter system. Today's pacemakers have circuitry, which allows the right signals to pass through and which blocks out irrelevant or misleading signals. When clinicians program the sensitivity settings of a pacing system, they are adjusting this filter system. (Note that making a sensitivity setting higher makes the device "less sensitive," while making the sensitivity setting lower makes the device "more sensitive." This can seem counterintuitive. Think of the sensitivity setting as the filter; when you set it high, you are allowing all signals up to and including that height to pass through. When you decrease the sensitivity setting, you are allowing only signals up to and including that height to pass through.)

The filter is the first line of defense against stray signals. When the device is only picking up the signals from the appropriate chamber of the heart, the actual signal that gets through may be fairly weak. A sense amplifier is installed to pump up the signal to make it large enough for the device to work with. Part of this system involves a comparator, a component used in many types of computer systems. A comparator compares the filtered and amplified signal against a baseline to size it properly. At this point, the signal enters the device's logic circuitry and is evaluated (Fig. 6.2).

The function of the pulse generator is to generate electrical output pulses. To accomplish this, every pulse generator contains a battery in its titanium case. In fact, the battery is the largest single element inside the device, taking up as much as 50% of the total "guts" of the device (Fig. 6.3). Most pacemaker batteries have low voltages, usually around 2.8 V. Since pacemakers sometimes have to deliver output pulses more than 2.8 V, they rely on a circuit called a voltage amplifier to multiply the voltage output. A voltage amplifier works by storing the electrical output until the right amount of energy is available and then releasing it.

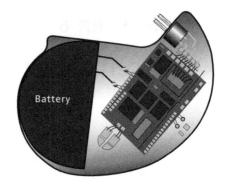

Fig. 6.3 Pacemaker can cut open, showing large section of battery.

When pacemakers were first invented, a variety of different batteries were used. In the early days, there were even nuclear pacemakers (Fig. 6.4)powered by plutonium!

Rechargeable pacemakers were popular in the 1970s, and some manufacturers worked with mercury-zinc and nickel-cadmium batteries. Once the lithium-iodine battery was invented and tested in pacemakers, nothing else has been used. While there is a variety of pacemaker batteries on the market, all currently used pacemaker batteries are variations of the lithium-iodine cell.

The lithium-iodine battery creates electricity through a carefully controlled chemical reaction between the lithium and the iodine. The internal re-

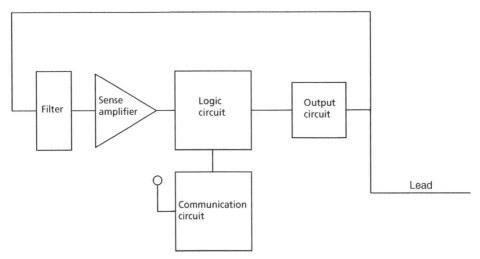

Fig. 6.2 Simplified circuit diagram of a pacemaker.

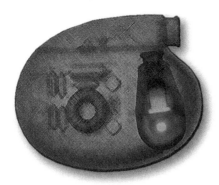

Fig. 6.4 Nuclear pacemaker from the 1970s. Using expensive and radioactive energy sources, they offered very long service lives. Some of the thousands of nuclear pacemakers implanted in the 1970s may still be in operation.

sistance of the cell increases as the battery depletes. A fresh lithium-iodine battery in a pacemaker is classified as having 2.8 V and about 10 000 Ω resistance. The battery is considered depleted at 1.8 V and 40 000 Ω. When the cell is *c*. 2.0–2.2 V with 20 000–30 000 Ω impedance, an indicator is usually given that the battery is nearing depletion and pacemaker replacement surgery should be scheduled. Many pacemakers today will report battery status on the programmer during a routine interrogation. Older pacemakers can be checked at follow-up by observing whether any indicators of depleting battery are shown (sometimes called "elective replacement" or "recommended replacement" or even the more severe "end of service").

One of the great benefits of the lithium-iodine battery over other sorts of power sources is that it depletes over a predictable and reliable course. It is not prone to sudden depletion or abrupt variations. The actual longevity of a pulse generator, however, depends not only on the battery, but also on how much it is used, which is why most manufacturers who state longevity figures are careful to add that they are projections based on a variety of variables. The actual longevity of any device depends on how often it paces and at what settings.

Every battery has some level of housekeeping current, i.e. the amount of energy it uses just sitting on the shelf. Even a pacemaker that never delivers a single output pulse will – over the course of many, many years – eventually wear out its battery. Housekeeping current is low in lithium-iodine batteries (usually < 1% per year), but the amount of quies-

cent current drain (as the engineers call it) depends in part on the device's circuitry. At any rate, it is not a major factor in overall device longevity.

Other minor factors that play a role in device longevity include the efficiency of the circuits of the device (do they waste energy?) and the impedance of the lead system. A high-impedance lead uses less energy than a low-impedance lead, which may save a significant amount of battery energy over a period of years. As a rule of thumb, standard lead impedance is usually stated as a range that can go from about 500 to 2500 Ω. Leads with higher impedance values probably save battery energy, while leads with lower impedance values likely use more battery energy.

But the single most important element in device longevity is pacing itself: how often does the device deliver output pulses and how much energy is delivered per output? A patient who requires virtually non-stop pacing will use up battery energy much more quickly than a patient whose pacemaker works only occasionally. Since this factor is not under physician or manufacturer control, most manufacturers state longevity projections based on 100% pacing, i.e. pacing every beat. This is probably extreme, at least for most patients, and can be considered a "maximum case scenario." Some manufacturers also state longevity projections based on 50% or some other percentage of pacing to give clinicians a more realistic life expectancy for the device.

The size of the output pulse is the biggest controllable factor in device longevity. The pacing output pulse is defined by two specific and programmable variables: the pulse amplitude, measured in volts, and the pulse width or pulse duration, measured in milliseconds. The pulse amplitude defines how high the pulse is, in other words, how many volts are being used. The pulse width determines how long the output is delivered. Taken together, they create a formula for how much energy is drained off the battery to deliver an output pulse (Fig. 6.5). Of these two variables (pulse amplitude and pulse width), the pulse amplitude or voltage setting determines the lion's share of how much energy goes into an output pulse.

It makes sense: a pacemaker that is pacing at 3 V per output pulse is using up more battery energy than a similar pacemaker pacing the same amount of time but using only 2 V per output pulse.

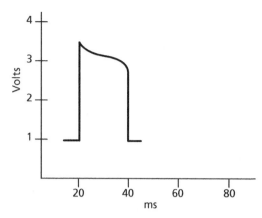

Fig. 6.5 An output pulse is defined by its pulse amplitude or height (measured in V) and its pulse duration or width (measured in ms).

Since output is such a crucial factor in device longevity, clinicians have to be very careful to program the output settings as low as possible, but not so low that they do not reliably do the job of pacing the heart. An output pulse has to be sufficiently powerful enough to "capture" the heart, i.e. to cause the heart to contract. A very small amount of electrical energy will not cause the heart to beat. The goal of every good pacemaker clinician is to find the "pacing threshold," the minimum amount of energy required to reliably capture the heart. Below the pacing threshold, the output pulse will not cause the heart to contract.

The problem with the pacing threshold is that it is an imprecise and individual setting. The pacing threshold of one patient is not necessarily the same as that of another patient. What is more, pacing thresholds are known to change within a single patient, even over the course of the day and can alter significantly over time. Many factors can affect the pacing threshold, and the biggest influences – drugs and disease progression – are more common in the pacemaker set than the general population. As a result, just because a clinician can determine a value for the pacing threshold of an individual today does not mean that the pacemaker should be set at that value. If that particular pacing threshold was taken at the "low point" of the day, it may not work well when the person experiences natural circadian changes in his pacing threshold. Furthermore, many pacemaker patients are seen only quarterly or half-

yearly. How can a pacing threshold set today be sure to capture the heart reliably 3 or 6 months later?

Clinicians have used a simple measure to accommodate these threshold variations called a "safety margin." As a rule of thumb, the clinician determines the pacing threshold and then doubles it. There are more scientific ways to discuss the pacing threshold and the safety margin: some physicians can chart a strength–duration curve and point to a specific spot on it – the rheobase – which marks the individual pacing threshold of the patient. The rheobase is then doubled to arrive at a point called the chronaxie, well within the limits of the strength–duration curve (Fig. 6.6). This mathematical approach relies on the same theory as the old rule of thumb: find the pacing threshold and double it. (Today, some programmers will map out a strength–duration curve for doctors to help them better visualize the difference between the pacing threshold and the recommended output settings.)

When a pacemaker lead is implanted into the heart, the pacing threshold is measured intraoperatively. The pacing threshold is the lowest amount of energy that is required to consistently cause depolarization of the heart. Almost immediately, and for several weeks thereafter, the lead goes through an acute-to-chronic threshold change. This changing threshold is directly related to lead maturation and encapsulation of the lead at the myocardial–lead interface. The effect of this encapsulation is an increase in the amount of energy required to cause depolarization. Historically, this increase was reported to be as much as five- to 10-fold! With today's new lead technology and the use of steroid-eluting leads, this threshold change is more likely to be two- to threefold.

In addition to the acute-to-chronic threshold change, the stimulation threshold can and will change from day to day. These changes are caused by factors such as electrolytic imbalance, acid-base changes, activity levels, drugs, eating, and many others. The problem with changing thresholds is that they are unpredictable. Therefore, in clinical procedure, physicians are forced to set a large safety margin – which can translate that they waste energy to promote safety.

What this means to the clinician is that most pacemakers are programmed to deliver considerably more energy than is probably needed. The idea

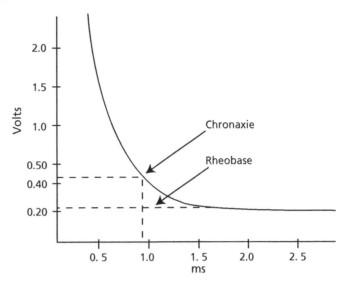

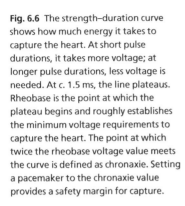

Fig. 6.6 The strength–duration curve shows how much energy it takes to capture the heart. At short pulse durations, it takes more voltage; at longer pulse durations, less voltage is needed. At c. 1.5 ms, the line plateaus. Rheobase is the point at which the plateau begins and roughly establishes the minimum voltage requirements to capture the heart. The point at which twice the rheobase voltage value meets the curve is defined as chronaxie. Setting a pacemaker to the chronaxie value provides a safety margin for capture.

is that it is better to err on the side of safety, since there is very little point to a pacemaker that is unable to capture and pace the heart. By setting the safety margin so high, physicians have confidence that the heart will be paced – but considerable battery energy is wasted in the process.

An interesting new algorithm in some pacemakers today allows physicians to avoid programming a wasteful safety margin without compromising the pacing therapy needed by the patient. These algorithms – which will be discussed more in a later chapter – assess the pacing threshold regularly and then deliver an output that is large enough to capture the heart. By matching the patient's ever-changing pacing threshold to the device output, the device does not have to deliver large output pulses to capture the heart. These algorithms have added many years longevity to the average pacemaker. In fact, today's pacemakers are smaller than ever before but last much longer! It is not unusual to see projected longevity values for pacemakers of as high as 10 years or more.

The pacemaker holds its sophisticated components, filters, memory, and other computer elements on a small board known as a "hybrid," so named because it contains a mixture of different types of components on a single, small flat board.

Next to the hybrid is a battery, which occupies most of the space in the device housing. The hybrid and battery are contained by a titanium metal case that is laser-welded together and hermetically sealed to keep body fluids from infiltrating the pacemaker

components. Titanium is the optimal metal for the pacemaker housing because it is extremely light, stronger than steel, and biocompatible.

On top of the titanium housing (sometimes called a "case" or a "can") is a clear epoxy connector block. The block contains ports in which the lead or leads are plugged. A single-chamber pacemaker will have one port (for one lead for one chamber) while a dual-chamber pacemaker will have two ports (one for the atrial lead, the other for the ventricular lead). The new CRT devices will have at least three ports, since they need a right ventricular lead, a left ventricular lead, and an atrial lead for the pacing function. Thus, you can tell if a device is single-chamber or dual-chamber or a CRT device just by looking at it (Fig. 6.7).

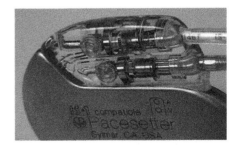

Fig. 6.7 Connector block or header of a pacemaker. The connector is made of clear epoxy. The two ports indicate that this is a dual-chamber pacemaker and requires two leads. Single-chamber pacemakers have one port and CRT devices have three ports.

The clear epoxy header usually has some sort of mechanism to secure the inserted lead in place. Some older pacemakers used a push-button connector, but others now use set-screws that have to be manually tightened once the lead is in the connector (Fig. 6.8). Although mechanisms vary, the end result is that the lead is inserted into the port, held securely, and somehow makes electrical contact. Tiny wires from this point of contact in the connector block go down through the case and into the device, a mechanism is known as a "feed-through," which allows a hermetically sealed device to receive signals from an outside source and to transmit output pulses out through the lead.

Pacemakers have an internal switch, which is activated when a magnet is placed over the implanted device. In older devices, a "reed switch" was used (Fig. 6.9) but newer systems use a giant magneto resistive or GMR. Regardless of which type of component is used, when a magnet is applied over the implanted device, the magnet circuit closes, and the pacemaker exhibits different behavior (usually called "magnet mode" or "magnet behavior").

Electromagnetic fields (EMFs) can influence pacemakers and other implantable devices. EMFs are present everywhere and generally are stronger close to the source as the electromagnetic force dissipates with distance. While many sources of EMF are known, the strength of these forces can vary dramatically, e.g. some household appliances generate very low-level amounts of electromagnetic energy, while other similar appliances may generate much higher levels. For this reason, sometimes people

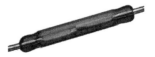

Fig. 6.9 A reed switch is a thin metallic strip within the pulse generator that can be manipulated by a magnet. Sometimes very strong electromagnetic fields can influence the reed switch as well, producing undesired results.

troubled by the presence of EMFs may require a field investigation to measure and detect sources of electromagnetic interference. Not all sources of electromagnetic energy are obvious, e.g. EMFs are known to be produced by some underground power lines and in-store theft detection systems (Table 6.1).

When a pacemaker patient encounters an EMF, it may or may not be affected, depending on the strength of the electromagnetic interference. Usually, the patient will be able to find relief by moving out of range or turning off the source. This should not permanently damage the pacemaker, but it may cause the pacemaker to go into a backup mode, which requires a short programming session to restore normal operation.

Pacemakers will alter their normal behavior when in the presence of a magnet or strong magnetic field. In fact, applying a magnet over the implanted device will initiate so-called "magnet mode" or magnet behavior. Although magnet mode can vary by manufacturer and even device (manuals from all devices should be kept on hand to look up magnet mode), it generally forces the pacemaker to pace asynchronously, which would mean DOO mode (for dual-chamber devices) and VOO or AOO in single-chamber devices. Asynchronous pacing means – as the code indicates – that the device paces but no longer senses.

Some programmers rely on the reed switch or GMR to change programmed parameters. Although this is not transparent to the clinician, many programmers temporarily close the magnet switch (using a magnet in the programmer wand) while programming the system and then open the magnet switch once the newly set parameters are made. Not all programmers use a magnet in the programmer wand.

Magnet mode can be useful for testing device performance or for other temporary tests. Asynchronous pacing, however, is not always comfort-

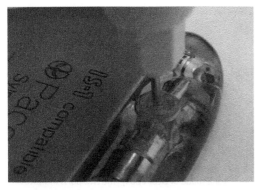

Fig. 6.8 A torque wrench is used to tighten a set-screw in the pacemaker header to hold the pacing lead securely in place in the header port.

Table 6.1 Some potential sources of electromagnetic interference

- Power lines (overhead and underground)
- Household appliances; can openers, blenders and vacuum cleaners produce stronger EMFs than ovens, ranges, washers, and dryers.
- Welding equipment, drills, machinery
- Electric blankets
- Air cleaners
- Office machines; electric pencil sharpeners produce stronger EMFs than copy machines
- Personal appliances such as hair driers, electric shavers
- Fluorescent lights

able or desirable for all patients. Many pacemakers nowadays allow the clinician to program the magnet mode to be "on" or "off." If magnet mode is programmed "off," even if a magnet is held over the implanted pacemaker, it will not revert to asynchronous pacing. This can be useful for pacemaker patients who are habitually troubled by encounters with electromagnetic fields.

Decades ago, a problem was sometimes encountered in which an older component called a reed switch got "stuck" or in which it could not be closed with a magnet, but these problems are now so rare that they can be considered almost "historical." Many clinicians who work regularly with pacemaker patients have never encountered such a situation, even once; however, any mechanical component can fail. In situations where a patient's device does not revert to magnet mode when a magnet is held over it, the first course of action is to reposition the magnet. Usually, the magnet is not in exactly the right place. Sometimes the magnet is too weak; two or three toroid magnets can be used, one on top of the other. Obese patients may require multiple magnets.

When in doubt about any of the device components, consult the manufacturer's sales representative, the manual for the device (manuals are now often online as well as being supplied as print editions), or call the technical support line from the company.

Further reading

Electrical And Magnetic Fields Research And Public Information Dissemination Program. Accessed from www.niehs.nih.gov on 20 November 2004.

Moses H, Moulton KP, Miller BD *et al. A Practical Guide to Cardiac Pacing*. Boston: Little, Brown and Company, 1983.

The nuts and bolts of pacemaker components

- Pacemakers contain mini-computers and batteries in a sealed titanium case with an epoxy connector block that links electrically to the inside of the unit by feed-throughs.
- Sensed activity from the heart is filtered, amplified, compared, and then used to help the device determine the heart's intrinsic activity.
- When programming sensitivity, it is the filter of the sensing circuit that is being adjusted. If the sensitivity value is increased, the device is made less sensitive. If the sensitivity value is decreased, the device is made more sensitive.
- All modern pacemakers are powered by lithium-iodine batteries because they are small, last a

long time, and deplete predictably.
- At the beginning of life, a pacemaker battery is *c.* 2.8 V and 10 000 Ω resistance. By the time the device is depleted, it will be at 1.8 V and 40 000 Ω. At *c.* 2.2 V and 20 000 Ω, a replacement indicator will appear on the programmer during follow-up sessions.
- Device longevity is impacted by many factors, the main one being the output pulse.
- The output pulse is defined by pulse amplitude (V) and pulse width (ms).
- The pacing threshold is the amount of energy the output pulse needs (V and ms) to reliably capture the heart (or cause it to contract). The

Continued p.42

Continued.

visual depiction of this is the strength–duration curve, with rheobase defining the minimum voltage needed to capture the heart and chronaxie (two times rheobase voltage, extended to meet the curve) as a reasonable safety margin.

- Pacing thresholds are individual and may vary over the course of the day as well as over longer periods.
- Most physicians establish the pacing threshold and then double it as the "safety margin" to make sure the output pulse is always sufficiently large to capture the heart.
- Some new pacemakers have special algorithms that assess the pacing threshold and deliver a precisely measured output pulse to save battery energy.
- When a magnet is placed over an implanted pacemaker, it closes a reed switch and forces the device into magnet mode, which is usually asynchronous (DOO, VOO, or AOO) pacing. When the magnet is removed, the device reverts to normal behavior. Some programmer wands contain a magnet since some devices require the reed switch to be closed during programming sessions.
- There are many potential sources of electromagnetic interference that may or may not affect pacemaker patients. Patients should be cautioned about likely sources and they should move out of range (or turn off the source, if possible) if they experience problems.
- Not all sources of electromagnetic interference are visible: underground power lines and in-store theft detection systems are just two "invisible" EMFs that can affect a pacemaker patient.
- Although any component can fail, problems with reed switches are very rare today.

CHAPTER 7

Lead technology

A lead is a specially manufactured, insulated wire that plugs into the implanted device and travels through the venous system into the heart. The lead forms a two-way path: it delivers signals (output pulses) *from the implanted device* to the heart and it transmits signals (electrical activity) from the heart back *to the implanted device*. A properly implanted modern lead can reliably perform these two functions for many years, even decades. While leads may seem simple, they form a crucial element of the pacing system. Unlike devices (which can be programmed to meet individual needs), there are many different types of leads available to the physician (Fig. 7.1). Implanting physicians select leads based on the device they will be implanting, the patient's anatomy, and their personal preference, usually based on the lead they feel has the best performance and handling characteristics; these judgments can be somewhat subjective.

Anatomy of a lead

The proximal end of the lead terminates in a con-

nector that plugs into a port in the implantable device. The distal end contains one or more electrodes that both send and receive signals to and from the heart. On the distal end is located some sort of specialized fixation mechanism, designed to help secure the lead in position within the heart. Between the connector at one end and the electrodes and fixation mechanism at the other, is an expanse of insulated wire, through which the faint impression of coils and cables may be seen. When properly in place, the lead connector is held securely into the pacemaker's connector header, while the distal end is fixated in the heart, to send and receive electrical signals (Fig. 7.2).

Fixation mechanism

Long-term performance of a pacing system depends on a stable lead position within the heart. Over the years, a variety of fixation mechanisms have been proposed to secure the lead in place with minimal trauma. These fixation mechanisms can be grouped

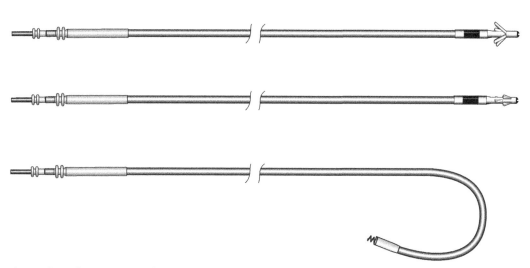

Fig. 7.1 Three of the many types of pacing leads include tined leads, finned leads, and an active-fixation atrial J lead.

The Nuts and Bolts of Cardiac Pacing, 2nd edition. By Tom Kenny. © 2008 St Jude Medical, ISBN: 978-1-4501-8403-8.

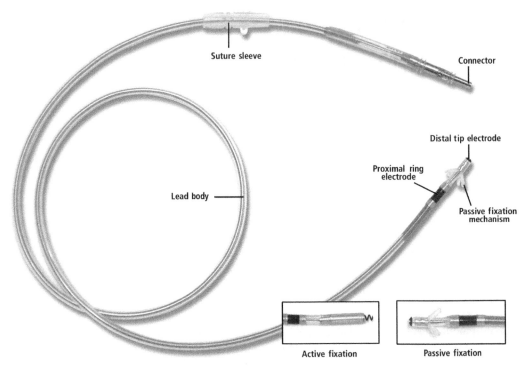

Fig. 7.2 Anatomy of a lead: the connector at the proximal end plugs into the pacemaker. The distal tip fixates in the heart using either a passive-fixation mechanism, such as tines or fins, or an active-fixation mechanism, such as a helix.

roughly into the active- and passive-fixation mechanisms, depending on whether the lead is supposed to attach itself within the heart (passive fixation) or whether the lead is screwed or otherwise fixed into the heart (active fixation). Historically, passive-fixation leads were more frequently used, but today active-fixation leads are becoming more common in clinical practice.

Passive-fixation leads rely on some sort of extension at the distal end that gets lodged in the trabeculae of the heart. These extensions vary in size, shape, and structure and may be called tines, fins, helices, or stabilizers. The most common passive-fixation lead used today is the tined lead. Typically used in the right ventricle, the tines of the lead catch in the dense trabeculae of the endocardium and give the lead some stability. During implant, the physician will test the lead for electrical signals and then gently pull on the lead to be sure it is firmly in place. In the event that the lead needs to be repositioned perioperatively for electrical reasons, a passive lead can be dislodged with slight force or twisting.

Once the lead is in place, a fibrotic capsule forms around it, which holds it very firmly in place. In fact, the fibrosis makes the lead almost part of the heart. This occurs for any chronic lead, whether a passive-fixation or an active-fixation model, and makes it very challenging to extract any pacing lead that has been in the body for a long time. There are risks associated with chronic lead extraction that must be carefully assessed before proceeding. The longer a pacing lead is in place, the more likely it is that complications will occur if the lead is extracted.

An active-fixation lead has a screw, hook, or helix that must penetrate the endocardial tissue to secure the lead. The most popular active-fixation lead used today is the extendable–retractable helix. With this lead, the corkscrew-shaped helix remains safely within the distal tip of the lead during implantation and venous passage. Once the implanting physician has determined the proper lead location, the proximal end of the lead can be manipulated to extend the helix out of its protective sheath. The extendable–retractable design was created in part to allow active-fixation leads to pass through the tricuspid valve without "catching." Once an active-fixation lead is in position, the helix is extended and screws into the endocarium, fixing the lead in place. The implanting team will then test its electrical values. Should the active-fixation lead need to be repositioned perioperatively, it can be "unscrewed" out of one location and then re-affixed with relative ease. Once the lead is permanently placed, a fibrotic capsule grows around the interface of the lead and tissue, securing the lead very firmly in place.

Comparing active and passive fixation

Passive-fixation mechanisms may be somewhat more common, particularly in right ventricular applications. They are relatively easy to implant and have a long track record of excellent performance. The passive-fixation mechanism on the distal end of the lead, however, increases lead body diameter and requires a larger venous introducer than comparable active-fixation leads. This could be a disadvantage for patients with small vessels, patients who need two or more leads in a vein, or for implanters who prefer to use the smallest possible introducer.

Active-fixation leads are slimmer, fit down a smaller introducer, but create a trauma at the point of lead–tissue interface. It has been observed that the fibrous tissue ingrowth covers a passive-fixation lead more quickly than an active-fixation lead; this means that, in general, a passive-fixation lead can stabilize and deliver good chronic thresholds more quickly than an active-fixation lead. Active-fixation leads are particularly important for use in the atria, where there are not as many trabeculae (Table 7.1).

While left-heart leads are outside the scope of this book, leads intended to pace the left ventricle have a characteristic curve at the distal end and no conventional right-heart type fixation mechanism.

Steroid elution

In the past decade, a major advancement in lead technology has been the inclusion of a small quantity of steroid (typically dexamethasone sodium phosphate) on the tip of the lead. Some leads place the steroid in a small core within the lead, while other lead designs allow for steroid in the form of a plug or coating on the tip (Fig. 7.3).

It had long been observed that pacing thresholds were initially quite low at implant, spiked quickly upward, then descended and plateaued at a level somewhere in-between (Fig. 7.4). The explanation for this acute-to-chronic threshold rise is believed to be inflammation at the site where the lead meets the myocardium. At first, there is no inflammation, so the pacing threshold is low. As the lead–tissue interface becomes inflamed, the threshold rises sharply. As the inflammation diminishes and scar tissue forms, the threshold goes down, but never back to its original level.

This threshold rise right after implantation poses clinical concern for setting the output values on the pacemaker. Output values that would work well at the low threshold value may fail to capture the heart at the peak, which is why generous safety margins are recommended when programming the output values for a new implant.

The drugs in a steroid-eluting lead minimize the inflammation and almost eliminate the initial threshold rise characteristic of non-steroid-eluting

Table 7.1 Comparison of active-fixation and passive-fixation leads

	Active-fixation lead	Passive-fixation lead
Lead diameter	Smaller	Larger
Introducer size	Smaller	Larger
Lead–tissue interface	Trauma	Atraumatic
Fibrotic ingrowth	Slower	Faster
Repositioning at implant	Easy	Easy
Right ventricular application	Less common	Very common
Atrial application	Very common	Very rarely
Proximal manipulation needed to secure lead	Yes	No
Chronic thresholds	Slightly higher	Slightly lower

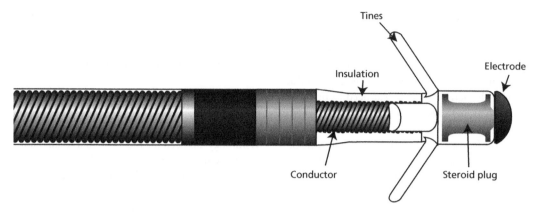

Fig. 7.3 Steroid plug on a steroid-eluting cardiac pacing lead.

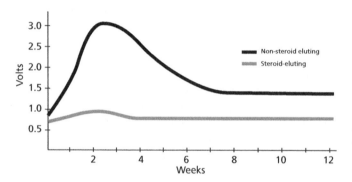

Fig. 7.4 Non-steroid-eluting pacing leads exhibit a low initial threshold, rise sharply and then plateau to a stabilized threshold value at around 6–8 weeks. Steroid-eluting leads remain at a relatively low, stable threshold value over the life of the lead.

leads. Patients who receive steroid-eluting leads experience less dramatic threshold changes as the system shifts from acute to chronic. The slow release of the steroid helps manage the long-term threshold.

While the clinical benefits of steroid-eluting leads have been established, the exact mechanism by which they work is not completely clear. When a steroid-eluting lead is used, the fibrotic capsule surrounding the lead–tissue interface tends to be smaller and thinner, but not to the extent that it would need to be to reduce the threshold by itself. For that reason, steroid-elution technology may advance in the future as we better understand how and why it works.

Electrode configuration

The function of a lead is to send and deliver electrical signals to and from the heart. To accomplish this, the lead relies on one or two electrodes at the distal end that connect to matching electrodes at the proximal end, which is plugged into the device.

In pacing lingo, leads with one electrode at each end are called *unipolar,* while leads with two electrodes at each end are *bipolar.* These terms are a bit misleading, since all electrical circuits have two poles: an anode (positive pole) and a cathode (negative pole). The difference is not how many poles the lead has (all leads have two poles); the distinction is where the poles are located. Unipolar leads have only *one pole on the lead itself;* bipolar leads have *both poles on the lead* (Table 7.2).

A unipolar lead uses its distal electrode as the cathode and takes the metal outer casing of the implanted device as the anode. This creates a large electrical circuit, which forms a corresponding large pacing artifact on an ECG. Because a unipolar circuit is so large, it may cause stimulation of nearby chest muscles. Unipolar leads rely on a simple technology that requires only one conductor wire, so they are thinner and more flexible than bipolar leads. They

Table 7.2 Bipolar and unipolar pacing leads

	Bipolar lead	Unipolar lead
Pacing artifact	Small	Large
Pectoral stimulation	Almost never	Possible
Myopotential interference	Almost never	Possible
Size	Larger diameter	Smaller diameter
Flexibility	Bulkier, stiffer	Thinner, more flexible
Reliability record	Excellent	Near perfect

enjoy an unsurpassed record of reliability and out-standing performance.

A bipolar lead uses the two electrodes on its distal end to form anode and cathode, creating a smaller, tighter circuit that produces a smaller pacing artifact and virtually no muscle stimulation. Since a bipolar lead must contain two wires or coils to conduct signals from both electrodes, it is often thicker, bulkier, and may be less flexible than a comparable unipolar lead. Recent advances in bipolar lead technology have created new bipolar pacing leads that are actually thinner and more flexible than older unipolar models. New data suggest that modern bipolar leads are even more reliable.

When it comes to receiving signals from the heart, bipolar leads have a distinct advantage, in that they are much less likely to pick up stray signals or interference than unipolar leads. The body generates lots of electrical energy in the course of the day, including myopotentials, a type of "muscle noise" that the lead might detect. Myopotentials are more likely to be picked up by the larger unipolar circuit than the smaller bipolar circuit.

Electricity and electrode design

Without getting overly technical, it is important to grapple with some basic electrical terms to better understand why pacing electrodes are designed and shaped the way they are.

The electricity that flows through the pacing lead – either from signals picked up in the heart and being forwarded to the implanted device or electrical outputs from the device traveling to the myocardial tissue – is known to engineers as "current." Anything that opposes the normal flow of current is called "impedance." The best way we have of measuring electricity is in terms of voltage, which is defined as the product of current times impedance.

For pacing experts, the most quoted mathematical formula is Ohm's law, generally stated $V = IR$, where V is voltage, I is current, and R is resistance. While electrical engineers and physicists make a distinction between resistance and impedance, for the purposes of pacing and Ohm's law, resistance and impedance are the same thing. A more useful way of expressing Ohm's law is $I = V/R$.

From Ohm's law, it has been determined that *the lower the resistance, the greater the current flow*. Conversely, the higher the resistance, the lower the current flow. Since current flow relates to the amount of power that the pacemaker drains from the battery, this resistance value – known in pacing universally (if somewhat incorrectly) as "impedance" – becomes an important predictor of device longevity. *A low impedance value means the device is able to deliver more current or electricity.* Low impedance is efficient for the pacemaker.

While relatively low impedance is a good thing for the pacemaker, *the electrode itself benefits from a high impedance value*, since high impedance reduces the amount of current flowing through it, and thus saves energy. For that reason, high-impedance electrodes (sometimes called high-impedance leads) are generally advertised as being of special benefit, because the high impedance at the electrode surface spares a lot of energy and does not prematurely drain the battery.

When it comes to impedance, it is good for a pacemaker to have low impedance and it is good for a lead (or electrode) to have high impedance.

Engineers know that the best way to increase impedance on the surface of an electrode is to reduce its overall diameter; the smaller the electrode, the higher the impedance (Fig. 7.5).

Impedance values can be thought of as the sum of all forces opposing the flow of current in the electronic circuit. Generally, lead impedance for a pacing lead will fall into the range of 300–1500 Ω. Lead impedance cannot be programmed and will vary slightly. However, any significant change (200 Ω or more) in lead impedance value over time can be indicative of a failure in the pacing system. Even a less dramatic change in impedance values over time can be a signal of an impending lead problem.

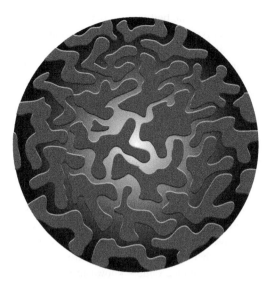

Fig. 7.5 Impedance varies based on the size of the electrode surface area. A large electrode surface area will cause thresholds to decrease and impedance and polarization to increase. To derive the benefits of a large surface area without increasing the electrode's circumference significantly, many electrodes today have a textured tip which increases surface area without increasing circumference. This is a magnification of a lead tip.

Another electrical factor that affects pacing leads is polarization, which describes the predictable flow pattern of charged ions in an electrical system. When a pacing pulse is emitted, the cathode will attract the positive ions and repel the negative ones. Ions build up over time. Over a length of time, this ionic build-up can affect and even block the flow of other ions, making it difficult for electricity to flow efficiently. More and more voltage may be needed to counteract polarization (Fig. 7.6). Electrical engineers have determined that polarization is related to the surface area of an electrode; *the larger the surface area, the lower the polarization.*

This left engineers of pacing leads with the dual challenge of creating an electrode that was very small (to increase impedance), yet with a large surface area (to reduce polarization). Modern lead technology has solved this puzzle by designing electrodes that are small in overall diameter, but have a textured surface to create a relatively large overall surface area.

Electrodes are typically made from platinum-iridium, Elgiloy (a special alloy), platinum coated with titanium, platinum, and iridium oxide (Fig. 7.7). These materials are biologically inert, resist corrosion, and have excellent conduction properties.

Conductors

The electrode on a lead connects back to the device through a wire known as the conductor. Once it is implanted, the pacing lead is subject to considerable mechanical stress within the body, because the heart and the body move constantly. As such, the conductor has to be flexible – ideally quite thin – and yet resistant to metal fatigue. (Metal fatigue can cause even a strong wire to crack or even break as a result of constant flexing.) The multifilar (or multistrand) conductor has met the challenge of forming a conductor which is strong, flexible, yet resistant to metal fatigue (Fig. 7.8).

The multifilar design wraps multiple thin conducting wires ("filars") together for strength, redundancy, and flexibility. A unifilar conductor is a single coiled wire; bifilar and trifilar conductors wrap two or three wires, respectively. More advanced multifilar designs have used six conducting wires or more.

Most conductors are made from a nickel alloy known in pacing lingo as MP35N. Another commonly used conductor is the drawn brazen strand (DBS), which takes its name from a metallurgy

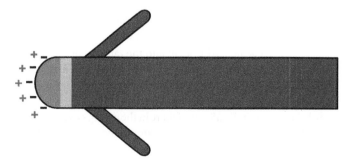

Fig. 7.6 Polarization at the distal tip of the lead is caused by the build-up of ions on or near the electrode.

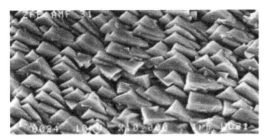

Fig. 7.7 Microscopic close-up of electrode surface area, showing titanium-coated platinum iridium used in some pacing leads.

technique. A DBS conductor uses MP35N wires and draws them together with heated silver.

A unipolar lead requires only one conductor wire (Fig. 7.9). (There is only one electrode on the lead to connect back to the electrode on the connector in the device.)

Bipolar leads need two conductor wires (Fig. 7.10). (There are two electrodes on the lead to connect back to two electrodes on the connector in the device.)

Over the years, engineers have proposed various mechanisms to allow a pacing lead to accommodate two conductor coils. In the earliest days of pacing,

the two coils were insulated and placed side-by-side in the lead body, making a rather fat bipolar lead. The next major design advancement was the so-called "coaxial bipolar lead," which put one coil inside the other, separated by a layer of insulation. Coaxial leads are thicker and less flexible than unipolar leads. Parallel-wound coils and thinner conductor wires have created modern bipolar leads that are reasonably thin, flexible, and reliable.

Insulation

Pacing leads are insulated wire, and there are only two main types of insulation used by all manufacturers all over the world: silicone and polyurethane. Both offer distinct advantages and disadvantages. The implanting physician will often have a preference for one sort of insulation over another.

Silicone rubber, the insulation material used in the very first pacing leads, has a track record of 40 years of reliable performance. Silicone is flexible and easy to manufacture. However, silicone nicks and abrades easily. Once in contact with blood, silicone has a relatively high coefficient of friction, making it harder to maneuver through the veins.

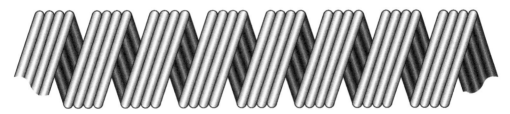

Fig. 7.8 Multifilar lead conductor.

Outer insulation   Coil (cathode)

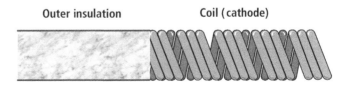

Fig. 7.9 Unipolar pacing lead with one conductor coil that serves as the cathode inside an insulated sheath.

Fig. 7.10 Bipolar pacing lead with an outer coil wrapped around an inner coil. The inner coil acts as the cathode, while the outer coil serves as the anode. The two coils are separated by a layer of inner insulation.

Outer insulation   Outer coil (anode)   Inner insulation   Inner coil (cathode)

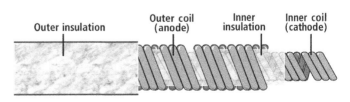

Polyurethane insulation was introduced later. With its greater strength, abrasion resistance, and lower coefficient of friction in the blood, polyurethane seemed like the perfect insulator. Unfortunately, polyurethane experienced some early clinical failures that tainted its reputation. These early failures related to a type of polyurethane known as P80A, which developed cracks and breaks that compromised the lead. We now know from subsequent investigations that these cracks were caused by environmental stress during the manufacturing process rather than damage that occurred to the lead while it was in the body.

The use of P55D (instead of P80A) and different manufacturing processes have greatly improved the performance of polyurethane leads. Even modern polyurethane leads may still exhibit microscopic cracks on the surface, but these are generally not of clinical significance. Thus, polyurethane is considered a safe and reliable insulation material that offers some advantages over silicone.

The clinical community has accepted both polyurethane (P55D) and silicone rubber as safe and effective lead insulation materials (Table 7.3). Today, there is even a new insulation material that employs both silicone and polyurethane in a blend that combines the best of both materials.

Connectors

The lead's proximal end is plugged into the pacemaker. In older-generation devices, a wide variety of connector pins were in use, complicating implants by requiring adapters. Recent standardizations have created connectors that allow most modern pacing leads to work with most modern pacemakers.

Because electrodes on the lead must connect with electrodes within the pacemaker, a bipolar pacemaker requires bipolar leads, while a unipolar pacemaker requires unipolar leads. Some bipolar devices allow the electrode configuration to be programmed (bipolar or unipolar), but bipolar leads are required. (A bipolar lead can function as a unipolar lead if the pacemaker allows it to be programmed that way; a unipolar lead, on the other hand, can only be unipolar.)

Modern pacing leads are built to accommodate the International Standard 1 (IS-1), which is a 3.2 mm diameter pin (Fig. 7.11, Table 7. 4). In clinical practice, older leads with longer pins, pacemaker ports with no sealing rings, and even 5 or 6 mm leads may be seen. In such cases, adapters can be used to allow these older-generation leads to plug into more modern devices. The representative of the lead manufacturer can assist in helping make the right connection for such systems (Table 7.5).

Atrial and ventricular applications

For implant in the right ventricle, most implanters prefer a straight lead, with either an active or a passive-fixation mechanism. When it comes to the right atrium – which is much smaller than the ventricle and has smooth, thin walls – many implanters prefer an active-fixation mechanism and a lead that is somewhat curved to get a better position in the atrium.

For this reason, many physicians prefer to use a specially configured atrial J lead for right atrial application. The J shape is preformed in the lead itself. During implant, the physician places a stiff stylet into the lead, which temporarily straightens the lead for venous pas-

Table 7.3 Silicone rubber and polyurethane lead insulation

	Silicone rubber	Polyurethane
Track record	Longer	Shorter
Tear strength	Weaker	Stronger
Flexibility	Greater	Lesser
Cuts, tears, abrasion	More likely	Less likely
Friction in blood	Greater	Less
Flexibility	More flexible	Stiffer
Manufacturing	Easy	More complicated
Environmental stress cracking	Not susceptible	May be susceptible
Metal ion oxidation	Not susceptible	Susceptible; don't use with silver
Reputation	Good; long track record	Suffered setback with early P80A failures; newer

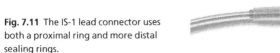

Fig. 7.11 The IS-1 lead connector uses both a proximal ring and more distal sealing rings.

Sealing rings

Terminal pin

Proximal ring

Table 7.4 Lead connectors and pacemaker connector standards

IS-1 (leads)	3.2 mm width, sealing rings, short pin, may be unipolar or bipolar
VS-1 (pacemaker)	Short aperture, may or may not have sealing rings
VS-1A (pacemaker)	Long aperture, no sealing rings
VS-1B (pacemaker)	Long aperture, sealing rings

sage. Once the lead is in place, the implanter withdraws the stylet and the lead resumes its J shape, allowing it to contact the atrial wall. The implanter then deploys the active-fixation mechanism, attaching the lead to the smooth atrial wall. All manufacturers offer an atrial J lead, and those on the market today have demonstrated safety and efficacy.

While left-heart leads fall outside the scope of this book, leads designed for pacing the left ventricle have a specially curved shape at the distal end to accommodate the challenges of accessing this side of the heart.

Lead lengths

Leads come in a variety of lengths to accommodate the needs of patients, who come in all sizes and shapes. Most manufacturers produce their main types of leads in several lengths. Pediatric leads for neonates are usually myocardial, meaning they are sewn onto the exterior of the heart (rather than passed through the veins into the heart) in a thoracotomy. Older children with larger veins get transvenous leads. In fact, these pediatric leads differ from adult leads only in terms of length. When a specific pediatric lead is not available (and there are very few on the market), the implanting physician will usually use the shortest available adult lead and wrap the excess around the pacemaker in the pocket. This technique also works on adults who may not need all of the length of the implanted lead.

Special leads

Nowadays, most pacemaker systems use transvenous leads, that is, leads that go through the veins into the heart. Rarely are other leads encountered in routine clinical practice.

A myocardial lead, mentioned earlier, is designed to be sewn onto the outside of the heart during a thoracotomy. Such leads were once commonly used for defibrillator implants, but are now mainly reserved for infants or in situations where a thoracotomy is being performed anyway. A myocardial lead requires major surgery to implant and is attached to the heart's exterior using some sort of patch or mesh material that is sewn onto the outside of the heart (Fig. 7.12).

Temporary pacing leads, also called "heart wires," are inserted into the veins and passed transvenously to the heart, and are connected to an external pace-

Table 7.5 Making the right connection. Will the lead type work with the pacemaker connector?

	IS-1	VS-1	VS-1A	VS-1B
IS-1 or VS-1 lead with short pin and sealing rings	Yes	Yes	Yes	Yes
3.2 mm lead, long pin, no rings	No	No	No	Yes
3.2 mm "Cordis" type lead, long pin, sealing rings	No	No	Yes	Yes

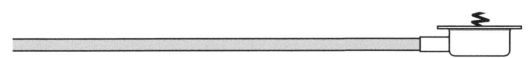

Fig. 7.12 Myocardial lead, which is implanted in a thoracotomy. The lead is sewn onto the exterior of the heart.

maker. Heart wires do not require precise positioning, since the external pacemaker can transmit higher energy output pulses without depleting its service life. Thus, heart wires do not need to be carefully positioned in the heart to gain maximum electrical advantage. A temporary pacemaker is just what it sounds like: it is used for a very short duration, typically during a hospital stay. The heart wires are completely removed before the patient is discharged.

Lead innovations

There have been numerous innovations to the pacing lead since the first transvenous wires were introduced. Steroid elution (discussed earlier) has done much to flatten out the initial threshold rise as relatively low acute thresholds gave way to significantly higher chronic thresholds.

New types of electrodes have helped make leads better able to "hear" what's going on in the heart and to distribute energy from the pacing output pulse effectively.

When it comes to lead insulation, for decades the main materials used were either silicone or polyurethane. Each insulation material had its own specific strengths (and weaknesses), and most pacing doctors developed a personal preference for one material over the other. Silicone tends to be more flexible and easy to maneuver, but it can abrade easily and two silicone leads can stick rather than slide against each other. Polyurethane is very durable and robust, and two polyurethane leads will slide well against each other, but polyurethane can be more rigid and some types of this material have been associated with stress cracking. Recently a new insulation material has been introduced, which is actually a mixture of both polyurethane and silicone in an effort to blend the best of both materials.

Another interesting advance in atrial leads occurred recently when a new bipolar atrial lead was introduced to the market with a 1.1 mm tip-to-ring electrode spacing. Research found that for bipolar atrial leads, the 1.1 mm distance between the two electrodes (which creates the antenna that picks up signals from the atrium) showed optimal characteristics. This new lead has been shown to reduce far-field R-wave spacing and to minimize oversensing problems. Far-field R-wave sensing occurs when the atrial lead picks up signals that actually come from the ventricle, but inappropriately attributes them to the atrium. It is interesting that this important innovation in atrial leads was created without any fancy new algorithm or new material; it was simply a new design that spaced bipolar electrodes slightly differently. This particular atrial bipolar lead handles and otherwise functions like a conventional atrial bipolar lead.

Further reading

Arnsbo P, Moller M. Updated appraisal of pacing lead performance from the Danish Pacemaker Registry: the reliability of bipolar pacing leads has improved. *PACE* 2000; **23**: 1401–6.

Byrd CL, Wilkoff BL, Love CJ *et al.* Intravascular extraction of problematic or infected permanent pacemaker leads: 1994–1996. US Extraction Database MED Institute. *PACE* 1999; **22**: 1348–57.

Crossley GH. Cardiac pacing leads. *Cardiology Clin* 2000; **18**: 95–112.

Rhoden WE, Llewellyn MJ, Schofield SW *et al.* Acute chronic performance of a steroid-eluting electrode for ventricular pacing. *Int J Cardiol* 1992; **37**: 209–12.

Sharif MN, Wyse DG, Rothschild JM *et al.* Changes in pacing lead impedance over time predict lead failure. *Am J Cardiol* 1998; **82**: 600–3.

The nuts and bolts of pacing leads

- Pacing leads can be unipolar or bipolar. This describes how many electrodes they have on the lead.
- Pacing leads can have active-fixation or passive-fixation mechanisms on their distal ends. This describes how they attach to the heart.
- A unipolar lead is thinner, has a larger pacing spike, but may stimulate nearby chest muscles. A bipolar lead has a smaller pacing artifact, is rarely susceptible to interference, and does not cause pectoral stimulation.
- In general, implanters use active-fixation atrial J leads in the right atrium and passive-fixation (straight) leads in the right ventricle.
- When it comes to the pacemaker, low impedance is good. When it comes to the electrode on the lead, high impedance is good.
- Both silicone and polyurethane (P55D) are accepted as efficient insulators; polyurethane is slipperier (but had a bad reputation early on), while silicone is more flexible.
- Bipolar leads have two conductors, which makes them thicker than unipolar leads with one conductor. The conductors can be arranged one inside the other (coaxial) or wound parallel.
- Nowadays, lead connectors are IS-1 and most leads can plug into most pacemaker ports. Older systems were not standardized, and lead connectors came in a variety of sizes, with different pin lengths and with and without sealing rings. When doing a revision on an older system, a pacemaker representative may need to advise the clinician about adapting the old lead so it can plug into the port of a new pacemaker.
- In terms of function, there is no difference between an atrial and a ventricular lead. Some implanters prefer to use a J-shaped lead in the atrium, but shape is the only difference in that lead.
- Myocardial leads are special leads that are sewn onto the exterior of the heart. They require a thoracotomy to implant and are used rarely, e.g. in pediatrics or when a thoracotomy is being performed for another reason at the same time as a pacemaker is to be implanted.

CHAPTER 8

Implant techniques

In the early days of pacemaker therapy, pacemakers were implanted by cardiac surgeons and then followed by cardiologists and the newly emerging field of electrophysiologists (EP), who are experts at implantable devices for cardiac rhythm management. Of course, the first pacemaker patients received their devices in a thoracotomy, a procedure not often used today for device implantation. Today's smaller devices and thin transvenous leads have made pacemaker surgery a minimally invasive procedure that is routinely performed all over the world by cardiologists and EPs, some of whom may perform no other type of surgery. While it is possible to implant a pacemaker on an outpatient basis, most pacemaker patients are admitted to the hospital for the procedure, which is typically performed in a surgical suite or a cardiac catheterization laboratory.

A pacemaker implantation involves a team of healthcare professionals: there should be one or more individuals who can operate an ECG and help with imaging equipment. A nurse (who may also be the ECG expert) is needed for administration of medication during the procedure. The physician – who may be a surgeon, cardiac surgeon, cardiologist, or other specialist – performs the actual surgery. Most pacemaker procedures are attended by a representative from the device manufacturer, who serves a valuable role as expert on the behavior, functionality, and characteristics of the device. A pacemaker representative can be a great help should problems or questions about the devices arise or should a special adapter or other part be needed during the procedure.

Most patients receive local anesthetic and sedation; although confused, mentally unstable, or combative patients may require a light anesthetic. Patients should be well hydrated, with food withheld for about 8 h before the operation. A routine pacemaker implantation takes about 1 h, but an unusual anatomy or other factors may extend this duration.

Pocket preparation

The first step in the implant is the creation of a pocket which is adequately large to hold the device but not so large that the device might migrate. After the patient is properly anesthetized, a small incision deep enough to reach the pectoralis fascia is made approximately an inch below and parallel to the clavicle. Unless there are compelling reasons to do otherwise, the patient's non-dominant side is the preferred pocket site (most patients are right handed and would thus have a pocket on the left) (Fig. 8.1). Using blunt and sharp dissection, a prepectoralis

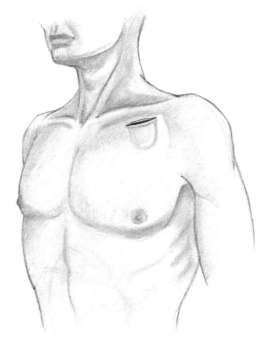

Fig. 8.1 The pacemaker pocket is typically in the upper chest on the patient's non-dominant side.

 The Nuts and Bolts of Cardiac Pacing, 2nd edition. By Tom Kenny. © 2008 St Jude Medical, ISBN: 978-1-4501-8403-8.

fascial pocket is created. Many physicians will place a sponge soaked in antibiotic solution in the pocket until the pocket is ready for use.

Today's pacemakers are cosmetically appropriate for most patients, in that they are relatively small and flat and will not protrude sharply from the skin. For certain female patients, in particular very young or very thin individuals, the pocket may be created in a retromammary position (Fig. 8.2). This procedure requires general anesthesia. For retromammary pocket placement, an incision is made in the inframammary fold (seen when the breast is lifted) down to the pectoral fascia behind the breast itself. The device is implanted behind the breast, and physicians using this technique may rely on a Parsonnet pouch or small polyester bag to hold the pacemaker. The retromammary technique does not allow the pacemaker to be palpated, but it can still be easily telemetered and replaced (using the inframammary incision). The scar and pacemaker are not visible. Retromammary pacemaker placement does not interfere with normal lactation.

Other pocket considerations may occur in pediatric, young, or very thin patients. In some cases, an abdominal pocket may be a preferred location for the implanted device.

Venous access

The next step in pacemaker implantation is positioning the lead or leads, which nowadays are almost exclusively transvenous. Patient anatomy, lead size, configuration, type of pacemaker (one or two leads), and physician preference all influence the selection of the vein. While it is possible to access the heart using the internal or external jugular veins, the iliofemoral vein, or an axillary approach, the most common sites of venous entry for pacemaker surgery remain the subclavian and cephalic veins (Fig. 8.3).

The most common technique to access the subclavian vein is the Seldinger technique, in which an 18-gauge needle attached to a 10-ml syringe (containing anesthetic) is introduced through the pocket incision. The needle should be inserted with the bevel side downward and then advanced slowly

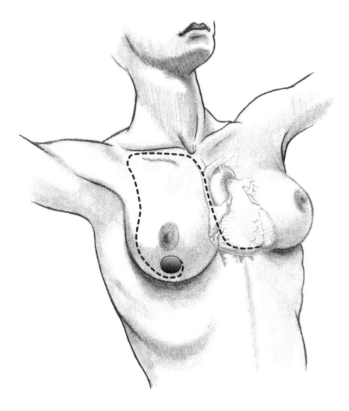

Fig. 8.2 The retromammary technique allows for pacemaker implantation so that the device and the scar are not visible. The device can be telemetered and easily replaced using the original incision.

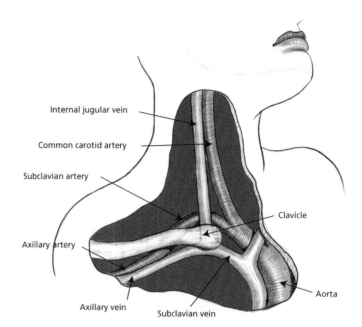

Internal jugular vein

Common carotid artery

Subclavian artery

Clavicle

Axillary artery

Aorta

Axillary vein

Subclavian vein

Fig. 8.3 Many different veins can be used for pacemaker implantation, with the subclavian and cephalic veins being the most frequently used.

along the tissue plane at the level of the junction of the medial and middle thirds of the clavicle and headed toward a point just above the notch in the sternum. Small amounts of anesthesia may be released as the needle moves forward. On reaching the clavicle, the needle's angle of entry is increased until the tip slides under the bone. Once under the clavicle, the needle should hold its course; changing direction could lacerate underlying structures. Negative pressure on the syringe should be used to check for blood aspiration, which would occur when the cephalic vein is punctured. Accidental arterial puncture is determined by the immediate presence of pulsing, bright red blood (remove the needle at once and apply compression to close the puncture).

The Seldinger technique is sometimes called a "blind subclavian stick" because the attempt to find the subclavian vein involves using a needle rather than a venous cutdown (which requires more surgical skill) (Fig. 8.4). There is a risk of injury with this technique. It is most effective in patients with normal subclavian veins. Repeated unsuccessful attempts to find the subclavian vein with the Seldinger technique suggest that the vessel is occluded or in an abnormal position. In such instances, another approach should be attempted rather than trying repeated blind sticks.

The Seldinger approach to the subclavian vein uses an 18-gauge needle with a 10-ml syringe and punctures the vein at the junction of the middle and

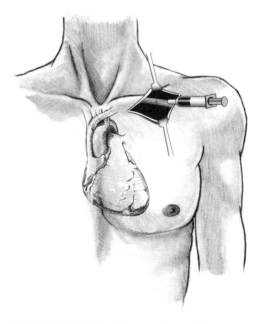

Fig. 8.4 The Seldinger technique can be used for accessing a vein for pacemaker lead implantation, when it is sometimes called the "blind subclavian stick" as the vein is accessed by needle rather than cutdown.

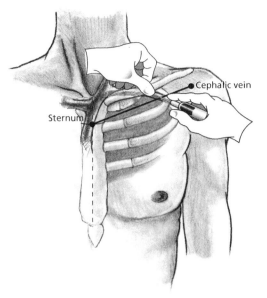

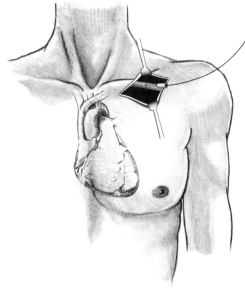

Fig. 8.5 In the Seldinger approach, an imaginary line could be drawn between the first rib and the clavicle for orientation. The needle is inserted at about the middle of the clavicle on this line.

Fig. 8.6 Once the needle has punctured the subclavian vein, the syringe is removed.

inner thirds of the clavicle. The landmarks for this venipuncture are the area between the first rib and the clavicle at the lateral edge of the sternum, described in a 40° arc (Fig. 8.5).

Once the subclavian vein is punctured (and confirmed by aspirating some blood into the syringe), the syringe is removed and an introducer guide wire is advanced through the needle and into the right side of the heart (Fig. 8.6). Fluoroscopy should be used to observe and confirm the advancing lead. It may take a few attempts to get the guide wire to advance into the proper place. When the guide wire is in place, the needle is removed and the introducer, the dilator, and the peel-away sheath are all advanced over the guide wire (Fig. 8.7).

Once the introducer is in place, the guide wire and the dilator are removed. A stylet is inserted into the pacing lead, and the pacing lead is now advanced through the peel-away sheath (Fig. 8.8).

Introducers are available in a variety of sizes, usually from about 8 French to 14 French (French is a measurement that defines the diameter of the introducer) (Fig. 8.9). The introducer size required depends on the lead or leads being used (most lead labeling will specify the size of introducer needed),

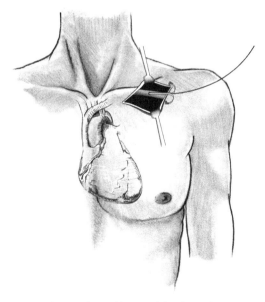

Fig. 8.7 The introducer, dilator, and sheath are then advanced over the guide wire. The guide wire and dilator can be removed, while the introducer remains in place until the lead is inserted. Many introducers can be peeled away at the end of the procedure.

and, as a general rule, the smallest introducer possible is preferred. When two leads are being implanted

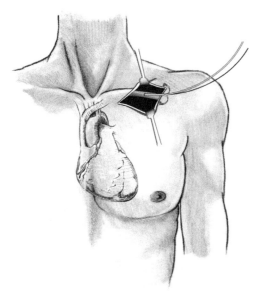

Fig. 8.8 A stylet is inserted into the pacing lead to give it some stiffness, and then the lead with stylet is inserted into the introducer and gently maneuvered under fluoroscopy toward the heart.

bust enough, it may suffice that the lead (with stylet inserted) be passed into the cephalic vein directly. Often, however, the size and shape of the vein warrant the use of a guide wire. The guide wire is passed into the cephalic vein and gently maneuvered into the right side of the heart under fluoroscopic observation. The introducer is then placed over the guide wire, just as was done in the subclavian approach.

In the cephalic approach, however, the guide wire is left in place as the lead (with stylet inside) is gently maneuvered into the right side of the heart. This approach is sometimes called "the retained guide wire technique."

The cephalic approach can be more challenging than the subclavian approach. It requires surgical judgment on the part of the implanting physician. When a standard guide wire is not successful, good results have been reported using a steerable hydrophilic guide wire inserted into the cephalic vein. One small study reported a 94% success rate with cephalic cutdown using a steerable hydrophilic guide wire.

(for a dual-chamber system) or when bipolar leads are used (which are thicker than unipolar leads), a relatively larger introducer is necessary.

Some physicians prefer the cephalic approach, which requires a venous cutdown. The cephalic vein is located in the deltopectoral groove, which is located between the deltoid and pectoralis muscles (Fig. 8.10). Although considered more of a "surgical approach" than the Seldinger subclavian approach, the actual surgical skills required are not extreme and the location of the cephalic vein is usually not problematic in most patients. Once the vein is identified, it should be exposed and a small incision made (Fig. 8.11).

The size and condition of the cephalic vein should be considered. If the cephalic vein is large and ro-

Fixating the lead in the ventricle

Lead placement always involves finding the optimal location for the lead in the heart with confirmation in the form of good electrical values. This involves knowledge of cardiac anatomy, dexterity in maneuvering the lead, good visibility of the lead on fluoro, and familiarity with the mechanics of the lead's fixation mechanism.

Once the lead has advanced to the superior vena cava, it should move relatively freely. At this point, if the stylet is withdrawn slightly and the lead moved back a bit, it can be deflected toward and across the tricuspid valve. If the lead gets hung up at the tricuspid valve, some physicians remove the straight stylet, curl a new stylet (usually by running it through

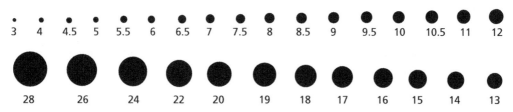

Fig. 8.9 Leads and introducers measure their diameters in units called "French." Introducers of 8–10 French are common in implants.

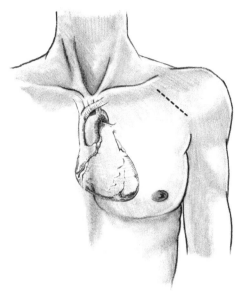

Fig. 8.10 The deltopectoral groove is the main landmark for accessing the cephalic vein with a cutdown procedure.

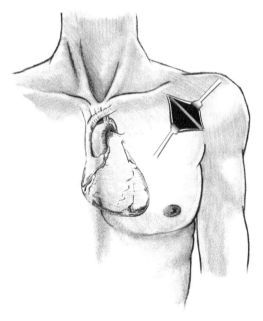

Fig. 8.11 The cephalic vein is exposed using a venous cutdown procedure. The vein is exposed and then a small incision is made to insert the guide wire.

a gloved thumb and index finger to impart a gentle curve; Fig. 8.12), and insert the curved stylet in place of the straight one. The curved stylet should remain in place until the lead is in the outflow tract; at this point, it should be replaced with the straight stylet.

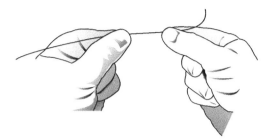

Fig. 8.12 If need be, a stylet can be curved by gently drawing it through gloved fingers.

Once through the tricuspid valve, the lead is in the inflow tract of the right ventricle. Fluoroscopy confirms the lead's position. As the right ventricular outflow tract is an anterior structure, a lateral fluoroscopic view will show a lead in the outflow tract to be in a retrosternal position. Most right ventricular leads are placed in the apex (not the outflow tract), but sometimes alternate placement sites – including the outflow tract – are desired.

Once a right ventricular lead is in the outflow track, slow withdrawal of the stylet will cause the lead to "fall" into the apex. Some additional directing may still be required to find the proper apical placement. Deep breathing by the patient causes the apex to descend into the diaphragm and may facilitate placement.

If the lead uses passive-fixation mechanisms, such as tines or fins, the lead will naturally lodge in the dense trabeculae in the right ventricular apex. Increasingly, physicians are using active-fixation leads in the ventricle, in particular with alternative sites (such as outflow tract or septum). In this case, the active-fixation mechanism (usually an extendable–retractable helix) is deployed to screw into the endocardium.

In clinical practice, electrical values of the ventricular lead are usually checked before inserting an atrial lead.

Fixating the lead in the atrium

Most pacemaker systems today that use an atrial lead are dual-chamber systems, meaning they require two leads. For that rarity – a single-chamber atrial system – the atrial lead is introduced using the subclavian or cephalic approaches described above.

When using a subclavian stick (Seldinger or modified Seldinger approach), two leads can often fit through the same introducer sheath into the heart (Fig. 8.13). This works particularly well when the subclavian vein is robust and the leads are relatively thin. A large introducer can accommodate two bipolar leads (for example, a 14 French introducer). First, the ventricular lead is introduced and stabilized in place; then the atrial lead is placed.

Another method of inserting two transvenous leads via the subclavian vein involves making two separate incisions (Fig. 8.14). First, a venipuncture is made and the ventricular lead is placed. Then a second venipuncture is made for the atrial lead. This dual-stick approach reduces the risk that one lead will dislodge the other, but it requires two venipunctures.

Another approach – the retained guide wire technique – can be used with either subclavian or cephalic access. In this method, one lead is introduced and placed. Then the guide wire is re-introduced (or never removed in the first place) and a new introducer is placed over the retained guide wire for the second lead.

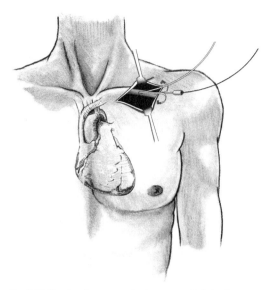

Fig. 8.14 Two leads may require two separate introducers. This allows the clinician to use smaller introducers, but requires two punctures.

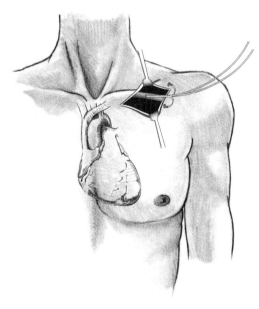

Fig. 8.13 One introducer is placed in the subclavian vein and both atrial and ventricular leads are passed through that single introducer. This requires only one stick, but it may necessitate the use of a relatively large introducer.

Atrial lead placement tends to be more difficult than ventricular lead placement, because the atrium is smaller, has thinner walls with less trabeculae, and may be surgically altered in some patients. The most common atrial pacing site is the right atrial appendage, but alternative sites are increasingly being explored and may be necessary for anatomical reasons.

Most leads selected for atrial use have a preformed J shape. A straight stylet is inserted in the lead to straighten it so that it may advance easily into the heart. When it reaches the mid-right atrium, as observed on fluoroscopy, the tip of the lead should be maneuvered toward the low right atrium. At this point, the straight stylet should be withdrawn about 10 cm, causing the J shape to form. The lead can now be drawn upward slightly into the right atrial appendage. On fluoroscopy, this will be seen as a medial and lateral motion of the J curve.

When implanting two leads, it is important to verify that the ventricular lead is not inadvertently dislodged by placement of the atrial lead.

Most atrial leads have active-fixation mechanisms. At this point, the screw-in mechanism should be deployed to affix the atrial lead permanently.

Intraoperative measurements

The intrinsic signal from the heart should be measured first. In rare cases, when the pacing threshold is tested before the intrinsic signal is measured, the patient can become pacemaker dependent. If this should occur, there is no underlying rhythm, making it impossible to measure sensing. In a pacemaker-dependent patient, no intrinsic signals exist to be measured. Acquired pacemaker dependency is usually of short duration. However, the whole issue of acquired pacemaker dependency can be avoided if intrinsic signals (sensing) are measured *before the pacing threshold is assessed.*

Sensing is tested by evaluating the signals that would make an intracardiac electrogram using a device called a pacing system analyzer (PSA). An intracardiac electrogram is similar to an ECG, except that an ECG is taken by measuring electrical activity on the surface of the skin, whereas an intracardiac electrogram is taken by measuring electrical activity from inside the heart itself. The amplitudes of the intracardiac signals are measured by the PSA to make sure they are large and strong enough to be picked up by the pacemaker. As a general rule, the intracardiac signal for the ventricle must be at least 5 mV and ideally between 6 and 10 mV in order to be useful. For the atrium, any signal > 2 mV is considered desirable.

If sensing signals are inadequate, the physician may decide to move the leads and test again. It is not unusual in pacemaker procedures to attempt more than one lead position in the search for optimal pacing and sensing thresholds. This process, sometimes called "mapping," is one of the most time-consuming aspects of the procedure.

In order to confirm satisfactory lead placement, electrical measurements must be taken before the leads are plugged into the pacemaker. These intraoperative measurements are taken using a hand-held PSA, which assesses pacing and sensing thresholds. A person skilled in using the PSA should take the intraoperative measurements.

First, the PSA should be programmed to a pacing rate that overrides the patient's intrinsic rhythm. This best mimics what will actually occur when the pacemaker is connected and pacing. The PSA delivers a pacing output pulse at a relatively high level of energy, and its effect on the patient's heart is noted on the ECG. This first output should capture the heart, that is, it should present on the ECG as a small pacing spike followed by a depolarization of the heart. The PSA then steps down the energy of the output pulse, lower and lower, until capture is lost. The value right before capture is lost is considered the pacing threshold. In other words, *the capture or pacing threshold is the minimum amount of energy required to consistently capture the heart.*

As a rule of thumb, pacing thresholds in both chambers should be < 1 V. Thresholds depend in large part on lead placement. Sometimes moving the lead even a small distance or repositioning it in the same area will have a dramatic impact on the threshold. Thus, if the physician feels that pacing thresholds are too high, he or she may decide to reposition the lead and test it again with the PSA.

Long-term performance is the key reason for spending the time intraoperatively to obtain good sensing and capture threshold values. It is well accepted in clinical practice that the larger the sensing (or intrinsic) signal that is obtained intraoperatively, the more likely it is that appropriate sensing will be maintained after device implantation. Also, the lower the pacing or capture threshold, the healthier the stimulated tissue. If you can stimulate healthy tissue with low energy, you are more likely to successfully capture the heart in the long term. The bottom line: healthy tissue puts out larger signals and requires less energy to be stimulated.

At this point, the PSA may also be used to measure lead impedance. Lead impedance values cannot be programmed and generally fall in broad ranges rather than specific values. But lead impedance values can be red flags for potential lead problems.

- *Low impedance* could indicate an insulation problem in the lead (such as a lead whose insulation was nicked or otherwise compromised during implant)
- *High impedance* could indicate a lead fracture, that is, a problem with the conductor coil of the lead.

Impedance values vary by lead type, so the labeling on the lead needs to be checked to define what is considered "high" and "low." Record impedance values at implant; impedance should be monitored with every follow-up visit. Large changes (either up or down) of 200 Ω or more suggest an existing or pending lead problem.

Connecting the device

Once the lead or leads are properly positioned, the pulse generator is removed from its box. The proximal ends of the leads are plugged into the ports of the pacemaker. The leads are fully inserted into the connector block and, depending on the type of device used, may be connected by tightening set-screws or otherwise securing the leads into place. The antibiotic-soaked sponge in the pocket is removed and the pacemaker is placed into the pocket. If there is excess lead length, it is then wrapped or hidden beneath the pacemaker in the pocket. Some pacemakers must be implanted writing-side-up, while others are not sensitive to this. (Check the pacemaker manual or consult the manufacturer's representative for information on the specific device.)

The pocket is sutured closed (Fig. 8.15). Usually, the patient remains in the hospital overnight and can be discharged the next day.

Further reading

Byrd CL. Safe introducer technique for pacemaker lead implantation. *PACE* 1992; **15**: 262–7.

Furman S, Hayes DL, Holmes DR. *A Practice of Cardiac Pacing*, 3rd edn. Mount Kisco, NY: Futura, 1993.

Gadhohe A, Roth JA. Retromammary implantation of an ICD using a single lead system: an alternative approach to pectoral implantation in women. *PACE* 1997; **20** (1 Part 1): 128–9.

Kistler PM, Fynn SP, Mond HG. The subpectoral pacemaker implant: it isn't what it seems! *PACE* 2004: **27**: 361–4.

Neri R, Cesario AS, Baragli D *et al.* Permanent pacing lead insertion through the cephalic vein using a hydrophilic guidewire. *PACE* 2003; **26**: 2313–14.

Parsonnet V, Roelke M. The cephalic vein cutdown versus subclavian puncture for pacemaker/ICD lead implantation. *PACE* 1999; **22**: 695–7.

Shimada H, Hashino K, Yuki M *et al.* Percutaneous cephalic approach for permanent pacemaker implantation. *PACE* 1999; **22**: 1499–501.

Sternbach G. Sven Ivar Seldinger: catheter introduction on a flexible leader. *J Emerg Med* 1990; **8**: 635–7.

Tse HF, Lau CP, Leung SK *et al.* A cephalic vein cutdown and venography technique to facilitate pacemaker and defibrillator lead implantation. *PACE* 2001; **24** (4 Part 1): 469–73.

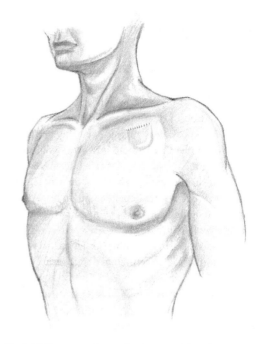

Fig. 8.15 The pacemaker pocket is sutured closed.

The nuts and bolts of implant technique

- While every patient is unique (and some may require unusual implant techniques), most devices implanted today use the cephalic or subclavian vein for transvenous leads.
- The subclavian vein is usually accessed using the Seldinger technique with a needle (blind stick).
- The cephalic vein is usually accessed with a cutdown technique (dissection).
- Other veins that can be used for pacemaker lead insertion are internal and external jugular veins, axillary veins, even the ileoformal vein.
- When a dual-chamber pacemaker is implanted, the two leads can be inserted through one incision or by using two incisions.
- Once the vein is incised, a guide wire is inserted. An introducer, dilator, and peel-away sheath are inserted over the guide wire. The guide wire is removed (except in the "retained guide wire

Continued p.63

Continued.

technique") and the lead (with stylet inserted) is maneuvered into place, as observed on fluoroscopy.

- The retained guide wire technique is used when two leads are being placed through the same incision. In this case, the guide wire stays in place after the first lead is introduced. The introducer, dilator, and sheath are removed. Then a new introducer, dilator, and sheath are placed and the second lead is inserted.
- A pocket is created for the device that should be just large enough to hold the device. For women concerned about cosmetic appearance and thin women, a retromammary pocket has proven successful.
- Once the lead is in place, intraoperative measurements of pacing threshold, sensing threshold, and lead impedance are taken using a PSA.
- The physician may decide to reposition the leads to obtain better intraoperative values.
- Always measure intrinsic values (sensing) intraoperatively before assessing the intraoperative pacing threshold to prevent acquired pacemaker dependency.
- The ideal pacing threshold during intraoperative

measurements is < 1 V; the ideal sensing threshold is 2–3 mV in the atrium, 4–10 mV in the ventricle. Lead impedance values are relative to the lead used, but high impedance suggests a lead fracture and low impedance suggests a compromise of the insulation.

- Healthy tissue puts out larger signals and takes less energy to stimulate. It is worth taking time during the implant to get the strongest intrinsic signals and the lowest capture threshold possible.
- Once intraoperative measurements are considered satisfactory, the leads are plugged into the pacemaker and the pacemaker is put in the pocket and sutured closed.
- Most pacemaker procedures take place in a surgical suite or cardiac catheterization laboratory under local anesthetic. Most patients stay in the hospital, but generally just for one night.
- It is not uncommon for a pacemaker manufacturer representative to attend the implant procedure and his or her presence serves to provide insight into device characteristics and functionality.

CHAPTER 9

Single-chamber pacing

Single-chamber pacing is based on the two fundamentals of permanent pacing: pacing (which means capturing the heart) and sensing (which means "seeing" the heart's own intrinsic signal). Without a solid grasp of capture and sensing, it can be impossible to sort through seemingly complicated pacemaker behavior. This chapter begins with these basic elements of cardiac pacing.

Capture

A pacemaker paces or stimulates the heart when it sends enough electrical energy through the lead into the endocardium to force the heart to depolarize (contract) in response. This depolarization in response to electrical energy from the pulse generator is called "capture" and it is the cornerstone of pacing.

Since the pacemaker output pulse appears on the surface ECG as a small vertical line called a "spike," it is easy to observe capture on a surface ECG or an intracardiac electrogram. This pacing spike is also sometimes called the pacing artifact. When a spike appears before a QRS complex, this indicates that a pacing output pulse was delivered, followed by a ventricular contraction – in other words, probable capture. Likewise, a pacing artifact right before a P wave means a pacemaker output was delivered right before an atrial depolarization – another likely case of capture.

One commonly used method is to watch for normal QRS conduction (in the absence of AV block, of course) at a consistent interval following each atrial pacemaker spike. Remember: during normal conduction, an impulse leaves the SA node, spreads through the atrium causing atrial depolarization, which is seen on the ECG as the P wave (Fig. 9.1). The electrical energy then crosses the AV node through the bundle of His to the left and right bundle branches and Purkinje fibers to activate the ventricles. This rapid spread of conduction through the intraventricular conduction system is seen as a ventricular depolarization on the surface ECG as the QRS complex. The normal QRS complex is narrow on the ECG, taking 0.06 to 0.10 s to conduct (60–100 ms).

In cardiac pacing, when the ventricles are stimulated by the electric impulse, the resulting QRS is wide and looks unusual. Therefore, ventricular capture is largely seen when the pacing spike is immediately followed by a wide (left bundle branch type) QRS (Fig. 9.2). This changed QRS morphology oc-

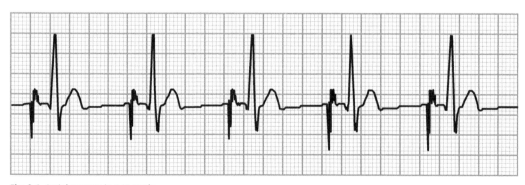

Fig. 9.1 Atrial capture in AAI mode.

64 *The Nuts and Bolts of Cardiac Pacing*, 2nd edition. By Tom Kenny. © 2008 St Jude Medical, ISBN: 978-1-4501-8403-8.

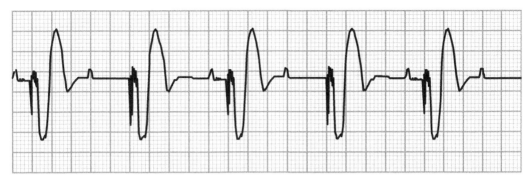

Fig. 9.2 Ventricular capture in VVI mode.

curs because the pacing lead stimulates the right ventricle first and then the impulse spreads through the septum to activate the left ventricle.

Atrial capture, however, is not as easily observed because the P wave amplitude is small on the ECG. Therefore, atrial depolarization as a result of pacing spikes can be more difficult to assess.

Failure to capture the heart can take a few different forms on a surface ECG. One of the most common is a pacing artifact with no resulting QRS complex or P wave. This indicates that the pacemaker delivered an output pulse but that it did not cause a ventricular or atrial depolarization.

Pacemaker programmers produce rhythm strips with annotations and other markers that help clinicians readily assess the meaning of the strip (Fig. 9.3). These annotations are reliable indicators of how the pacing system "interpreted" the various electrical signals it received. It is essential to realize that the device will annotate sensed events and mark when it paces, but it will not determine capture. Manufacturers use slightly different symbols and methods to annotate tracings, but these abbreviations and codes are designed to be intuitive and easy to understand, even without a manual.

A systematic approach is necessary whenever dealing with any pacemaker behavior, because there are many factors that can affect what the pacemaker is doing. Sometimes an initial strip or first impression can be misleading. For this reason, if a pacemaker output pulse (appearing in the form of a pacing spike) does not seem to cause a subsequent depolarization (appearing on the ECG in the form of a QRS complex or P wave), it should first be called "apparent non-capture." In other words, it looks like non-capture, but it is difficult to tell at first glance what is really going on.

Sometimes what is going on is "functional non-capture." This occurs when the output pulse of the pacemaker falls into the intrinsic refractory period of the patient. Each time the heart depolarizes, it takes a certain amount of time for the heart to recover electrically before it can depolarize again. This "waiting period" is called the refractory period. If

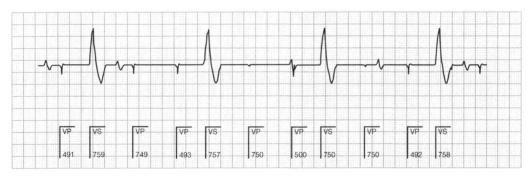

Fig. 9.3 An annotated VVI rhythm strip showing ventricular pacing outputs (VP) and sensed events in the ventricle (VS). Although the pacemaker records events such as AS VP (ventricular paced events), this strip does not show capture.

the pacemaker output is timed so that it occurs during the physiologic refractory period, the heart would be physically and electrically incapable of responding. Functional non-capture in a ventricular pacemaker occurs when the pacemaker spike appears in close proximity to the QRS complex. This can often be corrected by programming different refractory period settings.

There is another common reason for apparent non-capture. The pacemaker's output settings (pulse amplitude and pulse width) could be set too low to capture the heart. The patient's heart is capable of being captured by the pacemaker, but the device needs to be reprogrammed. This form of apparent non-capture can be easily rectified by programming higher output settings.

So how is output pulse energy best increased?

A pacemaker's output can be regarded as the delivery of voltage over time, i.e. a certain amount of electrical energy for a certain length of time. Increasing either of these (amount or duration) will increase the energy. For reasons of electrical economy, however, increasing the voltage has a proportionately larger effect on energy than increasing the duration. The electrical formula is described as energy = voltage(2) × time/resistance or $E = V^2 T/R$. This formula really means that *when you double the voltage, you quadruple the energy*. Doubling the time (duration) will only double the energy consumed.

The output pulse is regulated on the programmer by two programmable parameters: the pulse amplitude and the pulse width (Fig. 9.4). The pulse amplitude (measured in volts) literally defines how tall the electrical wave is. This setting is usually programmed to values of *c.* 1.5 V or 2.2 V or even 2.8 V. Most pacemakers only allow settings up to *c.* 7.5 V or possibly 10 V.

The pulse width or pulse duration defines how long the energy is delivered. This value is set in milliseconds, and is typically *c.* 0.2–0.8 ms.

Increasing either pulse amplitude (voltage) or pulse width (ms) will increase the energy of the output pulse. It is almost always more efficient (in terms of overall energy consumption and battery life) to increase the voltage (pulse amplitude) than to extend the pulse width.

During implant, the physician determines the capture threshold (also known as the pacing threshold). This is the lowest amount of energy needed to consistently capture the heart. Think of the pacing threshold as the bare minimum of energy needed to capture.

Capture thresholds are not fixed, permanent values. There is a change in the weeks immediately following implant and then fluctuations over the life of the pacing system. In the days before steroid-eluting pacing leads, every pacemaker went through a rather dramatic "acute-to-chronic threshold change." This sharp increase in pacing threshold was the result of lead maturation.

When a non-steroid-eluting pacing electrode is placed in the heart, an inflammatory process occurs. A fibrous capsule is formed at the "lead–myocardial interface," i.e. the place where the electrode meets the heart muscle. The tip of the pacing electrode actually becomes part of the myocardium. When this happens, the inflammation is replaced by lead encapsulation. The pacing threshold that was measured intraoperatively will now increase. Historically (i.e. with older pacing systems), this acute-to-chronic threshold change would take place in the first 2–8 weeks after implant. After lead maturation, the threshold decreases and stabilizes. It was not uncommon to see threshold increases of as much as fivefold over the intraoperative threshold.

With today's new pacing electrode materials and the introduction of steroid-eluting leads, this dra-

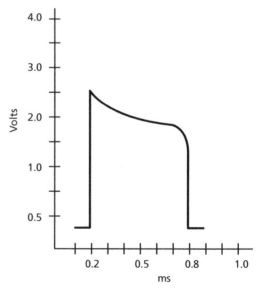

Fig. 9.4 The pacing output is defined by pulse amplitude or height (in V) and pulse duration or width (in ms).

matic increase has all but disappeared. A steroid-eluting lead may demonstrate a slight increase in pacing threshold in the period immediately after implant, but that increase is usually slight. Nevertheless, thresholds should be monitored closely during the first 6–10 weeks, as there can be wide variations among patients, even with steroid-eluting leads.

While the most well-documented pacing threshold increase occurs in the first few weeks after lead implantation, pacing thresholds fluctuate for many other reasons over the life of the pacing system. Pacing thresholds can change with medications and disease progression, two factors that occur frequently in typical pacemaker patients. They can also change with eating, posture, time of day, or just gradually over time itself.

To accommodate the fact that pacing thresholds are not static values and to assure consistent, reliable pacing, most clinicians use a simple technique to assure adequate pacing energy to capture the heart. The pacing threshold determined at implant or during follow-up may be regarded as the "bare minimum" of energy required to capture the heart. To assure pacing even when that "bare minimum" fluctuates, the physician adds a "safety margin." The safety margin is a "cushion" of energy that assures that even if the pacing threshold increases for any reason, there is still likely to be sufficient energy in the pacing output to capture the heart reliably. Typical pacing safety margins are 2:1 or 3:1, meaning twice or three times the capture threshold.

As a rule of thumb, a 2:1 safety margin is used for voltage (which has a more powerful impact on total pacing energy delivered) and a 3:1 safety margin is used for pulse width. For example, if a patient's capture threshold was 1.2 V at 0.2 ms, the safety margin could be 2.4 V at 0.2 ms or 1.2 V at 0.6 ms. Determining the actual output settings is a matter of clinical judgment and experience. Other factors – device longevity, medications, how dependent the patient is on the pacemaker – come into play.

The patient's capture threshold (which is another name for the pacing threshold) is likely going to be lower at the time of implant than at any other time. For steroid-eluting leads, there may be a very slight increase in threshold in the initial weeks post-implant; a much sharper increase will be seen in patients implanted with non-steroid-eluting leads.

After about 10 weeks, the pacing threshold levels off (it occurs much earlier with steroid-eluting leads but it can be safely assumed to have occurred with any conventional lead system at 10 weeks). After this point, the pacing threshold plateaus and remains relatively stable (with fluctuations) over time. Major changes in drug regimens or disease progression, however, can induce a major change in pacing threshold. Therefore, it is very important to assess capture thresholds at every follow-up session.

Many pacemakers and programmers offer automatic or semi-automatic capture threshold tests. The basic principle behind a capture threshold test is to pace in one chamber of the heart, gradually decreasing the output energy step by step, monitoring the ECG until non-capture is seen. The capture threshold is the value just before non-capture. For an experienced clinician with a modern pacing system, the capture threshold can be evaluated in a matter of a few minutes (Fig. 9.5).

Sensing

The other basic element in pacing is sensing, the device's ability to recognize the intrinsic activity of the heart. Sensing is vital to a pacemaker because it allows the pacemaker's internal computer to respond to the heart's own activity, which means that the pacemaker will inhibit pacing when it is not needed and the pacing will not compete or interfere with the patient's own rhythm. Since most pacemaker patients have intrinsic rhythm that prevails at least some of the time, sensing is a crucial function of the pacemaker.

The pacemaker senses through the electrodes on the distal end of the leads, located in the endocardium. When the heart depolarizes (contracts), it creates an electrical signal that the electrodes pick up and relay back to the pacemaker. To sense effectively, a pacemaker has to reliably sense the electrical signals generated by intrinsic activity. Of course, these electrical signals can vary in size (again, even over the course of a single day). Where and how the lead is positioned can change the size of the signal that reaches the electrode, and thus how viable the signal is for proper sensing.

Proper sensing can be observed on an ECG by noticing what is there and what is not there: if a prop-

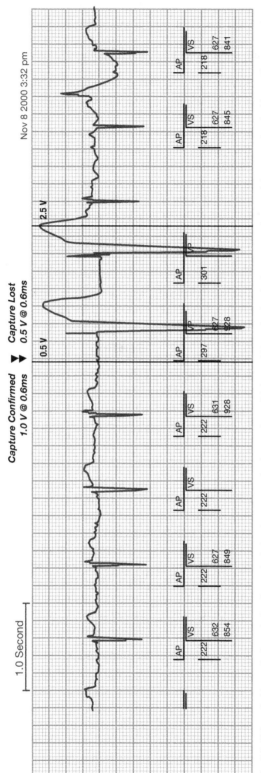

Fig. 9.5 Although this particular strip involves a dual-chamber pacemaker in a patient with intact AV conduction, it shows a stepdown atrial capture threshold test. The annotations show atrial paced events (AP) but in the center, the energy has been stepped down so low that these output spikes do not capture the atrium or conduct through to the ventricle.

erly timed intrinsic event and no pacemaker spike are seen, the pacemaker is most likely to be sensing appropriately (Fig. 9.6).

The two main challenges to sensing are "oversensing," i.e. sensing things that are not really there (or that should not be sensed) and "undersensing," which refers to not sensing things that ought to have been sensed.

Oversensing is usually seen on an ECG as inappropriately long pauses between pacing spikes. When a pacemaker suddenly stops pacing in its regular rhythm and there are gaps on the ECG where it should have paced, it often indicates that the pacemaker "oversensed" or sensed something that was not actually there (Fig. 9.7).

Although most clinicians work routinely with ECGs, it is important to remember that the ECG is not what the pacemaker "sees". The pacemaker relies instead on the intracardiac electrogram. An

EGM (as they are sometimes called) is similar to an ECG except that the signals come from within the heart itself rather than from electrical energy on the skin's surface. Many clinicians prefer to work with an ECG, which is usually available from a pacemaker programmer, which is probably just a matter of greater familiarity. While the ECG and EGM do correspond, remember that the pacemaker sees the intracardiac signal, not the surface ECG.

Undersensing occurs when there is an intrinsic event (P wave or QRS complex) that the pacemaker ought to have seen, but somehow missed (Fig. 9.8). An ECG with undersensing will typically show intrinsic activity followed closely by a pacemaker spike or intrinsic events that are not counted in terms of timing cycles. In such cases, the heart beats, but the pacemaker was unable to sense the electrical signal. An easy way to remember this is:

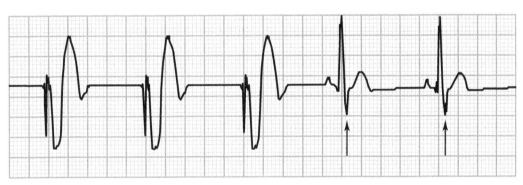

Fig. 9.6 Appropriate pacing and sensing in VVI mode. The arrows show intrinsic ventricular events at the proper time that inhibit the pacemaker (no pacing spikes).

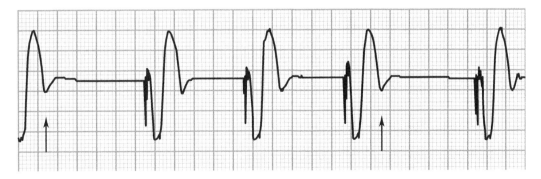

Fig. 9.7 Oversensing often shows up as pauses, in this case, the long distances between pacing spikes in this VVI strip. The pacemaker is oversensing, which means it is underpacing. In this case, the arrows point to low-level signals that the pacemaker has oversensed. In clinical practice, it is not always possible to "see" on the tracing the signals that a pacemaker oversenses.

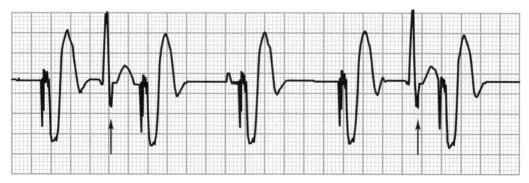

Fig. 9.8 Undersensing typically shows up as overpacing, i.e. regular paced activity in the presence of intrinsic activity. The pacemaker spikes and resulting ventricular depolarizations are evenly spaced, but the arrows indicate intrinsic ventricular events that the pacemaker failed to see. Had the pacemaker sensed these two events properly, it would have inhibited the next ventricular output pulse.

- oversensing leads to underpacing
- undersensing leads to overpacing.

When sensing problems are encountered, it's important first to recognize whether the pacemaker is not seeing what it ought to see (undersensing) or seeing things that should not be counted (oversensing). Sensing is controlled by a programmable parameter called sensitivity, which is measured in millivolts (mV). Sensitivity adjusts the device's input signals in such a way that it helps define the size of the signal to which the pacemaker ought to respond.

Although it may seem counterintuitive, increasing sensitivity (that is, making the device more sensitive) means decreasing the mV setting, while decreasing sensitivity means increasing the mV setting:

- to increase sensitivity, decrease the millivolt setting
- to decrease sensitivity, increase the millivolt setting.

Think of sensitivity as a wall. If you set the sensitivity wall at 2 mV, only signals larger than 2 mV are able to be seen over the wall. A 2 mV sensitivity setting means that the pacemaker will overlook anything behind the wall ($\leq$ 2 mV) but will see everything that pokes its head over the wall (> 2 mV) (Fig. 9.9).

If the sensitivity is reprogrammed to 4 mV, that raises the wall. Now only signals > 4 mV can be seen by the pacemaker (Fig. 9.10).

The highest sensitivity setting on most modern devices is *c.* 8 mV, but setting an 8 mV sensitivity value means creating a wall that is so high, very few signals will get over it. In other words, this high mV value makes the device very insensitive (Fig. 9.11).

While there are no energy considerations with sensitivity settings (as with output settings for capture), there is still a lot of clinical judgment necessary for setting the appropriate values for sensitivity. On the one hand, the device should be sensitive enough to sense and respond to intrinsic activity. Many cardiac signals are low-amplitude signals. In

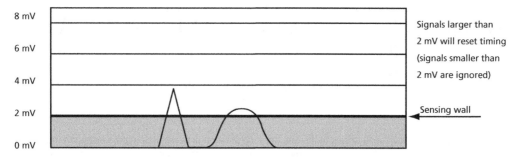

Fig. 9.9 Sensitivity functions like a wall. When it is set at 2 mV this "sensitivity wall" only allows the pacemaker to see signals that are taller than 2 mV.

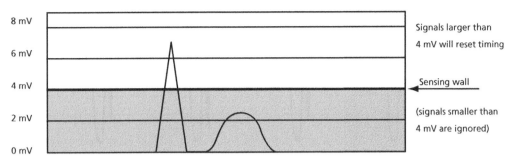

Fig. 9.10 If the mV setting is increased to 4 mV, this makes the device less sensitive. Now the only signals the device can see are those that are taller than the 4 mV wall.

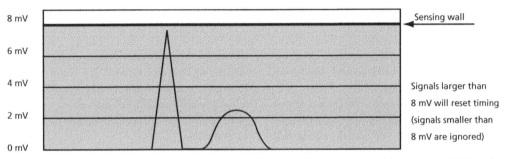

Fig. 9.11 Setting the sensitivity to 8 mV would almost never happen in clinical practice. In this case, the sensitivity wall is so high that only the very tallest signals have a chance of being recognized by the pacemaker.

fact, some arrhythmias may be characterized as having low-amplitude signals. Yet the device should be programmed in such a way that extraneous activity, muscle noise, or other electrical activity is tuned out.

Sensing is generally evaluated at the time of implant and then periodically assessed in follow-up sessions thereafter. The only way to evaluate sensing is to temporarily set the pacemaker to a pacing rate low enough to allow the patient's own natural cardiac activity to dominate; this is not always possible or safe for patients who may be pacemaker dependent or otherwise hemodynamically unstable.

For patients who can tolerate the device being temporarily inhibited, the pacemaker rate is set to allow the natural activity to come through and rhythm strips are checked for proper sensing function. The sensitivity can be reprogrammed and the new settings tested.

A clear understanding (and proper function) of capture and sensing is the first step in understanding various pacing modes. Pacemakers use a series of timing cycles to regulate their activity. When Earl Bakken bought a copy of *Popular Mechanics* to get the plans for an electric metronome to build his first pacemaker, he did it because he needed a precise timing mechanism. Pacemakers rely on accurately timed output pulses to mimic the heart's natural activity.

When a clinician programs the pacing rate of the pacemaker, he or she is actually setting the "pacing interval" or the "automatic interval" (Fig. 9.12). The pacing rate is programmed in pulses per minute (ppm), but the pacing interval is measured in milliseconds (ms). A conversion chart may be useful for calculations, but a good reference point is that 60 ppm (a common setting) equals 1000 ms (60 ppm means 1 pulse/s and 1 s is 1000 ms.) In the absence of sensed activity, the pacemaker set at 60 ppm will deliver an output pulse every 1000 ms or once every second on a rhythm strip.

As we know, pacemakers can also sense intrinsic activity. The time from a sensed or paced event to the next sensed or paced event is called the "escape

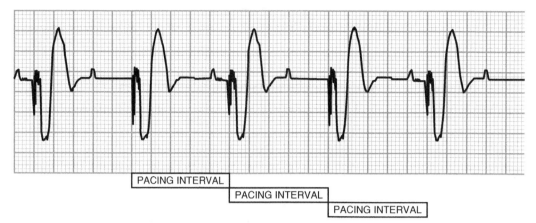

Fig. 9.12 In this VVI strip, each pacemaker spike (V) captures the ventricle. The V-to-V timing defines the pacing interval.

interval" (Fig. 9.13). Thus, if an intrinsic event occurs, the time between that and the next paced event is defined by the "escape interval."

To better understand how the pacemaker knows when to pace, especially in the presence of sensed activity, the timing cycles are actually subdivided into different phases. During the pacing or escape interval, there is a period of time during which the pacemaker can respond to sensed activity; this phase is appropriately named "the alert period." During this time, the pacemaker can sense and will respond to any incoming signals of intrinsic cardiac activity. For most devices, the longest component of the pacing interval is the alert period.

However, the pacemaker is not on alert for the entire pacing or escape interval. The reason for this is that there are many potential electrical signals that could confuse the pacemaker, such as:
• residual electrical energy from the last pacemaker output pulse
• the evoked response of the tissue, which can generate a lot of energy
• the T wave following ventricular depolarization.

To prevent the pacemaker from responding to these signals (and to prevent a ventricular output from pacing into a T wave), the pacing or escape interval has a phase known as the "refractory period." During the refractory period, the pacemaker will not respond to any incoming signals (Fig. 9.14).

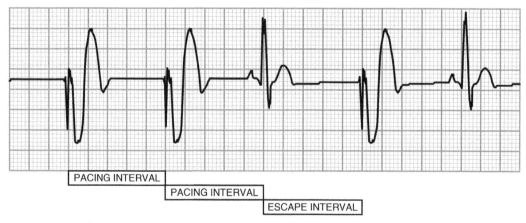

Fig. 9.13 The time from the sensed ventricular event to the next paced event is the escape interval. Except in the case of hysteresis (covered in another chapter), the pacing interval is the same length as the escape interval.

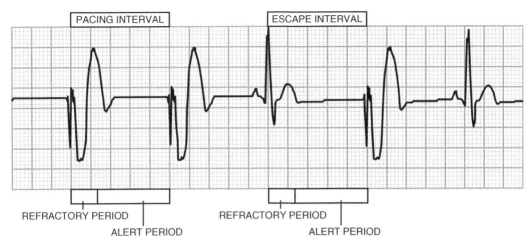

Fig. 9.14 This strip shows proper pacing and sensing in VVI mode. Sensed activity in the alert period will inhibit the pacemaker and reset the timing cycle. During the refractory period, the pacemaker will not respond to intrinsic signals.

(Note that pacemaker continues to "see" signals during the refractory period; it just will not respond to them.)

Pacing timing cycles are continually setting and resetting. If the automatic interval times out and no intrinsic activity is sensed, a pacemaker output pulse is delivered. This output pulse resets the timing cycle. If an intrinsic ventricular contraction is sensed before the timing cycle times out, the output pulse is inhibited and the timing cycle is reset (Fig. 9.15).

By far, the most common modes in single-chamber pacing are VVI and VVIR. Another way to see and understand typical VVI behavior can be taken from the St Jude Medical pacemaker manuals.

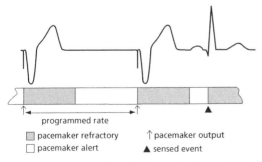

Fig. 9.15 A VVI pacemaker with alert and refractory timing cycles. A sensed ventricular event initiates the refractory period.

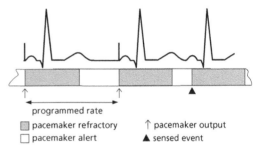

Fig. 9.16 Typical timing cycles for an AAI device. When an intrinsic event occurs in the alert period, it is sensed and initiates the refractory period.

Atrial pacemakers are considerably less common in clinical practice. The corresponding AAI diagram is shown in Fig. 9.16.

Triggered modes are used primarily for temporary diagnostic use or to avoid inappropriate device inhibition owing to interference (Fig. 9.17). A triggered mode paces when an intrinsic event is detected. The VVT and AAT modes use the same timing cycles, except that the response to a sensed event is a triggered output pulse (instead of inhibition, which is the VVI or AAI response).

Although uncommon, it is possible to program a single-chamber pacemaker to pace asynchronously, i.e. to pace without sensing. The VOO and AOO modes are shown in Fig. 9.18. In these cases, the device paces but has no alert period because it is programmed not to sense. Asynchronous modes are intended mainly for temporary use.

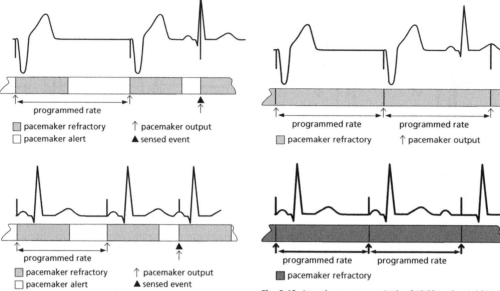

Fig. 9.17 Triggered ventricular (VVT) and atrial (AAT) pacing modes. A sensed event triggers a simultaneous output pulse and launches the refractory period.

Fig. 9.18 Asynchronous ventricular (VOO) and atrial (AOO) pacing involves no sensing behavior at all. The pacemaker delivers evenly spaced output pulses and is incapable of responding to intrinsic signals.

Although single-chamber pacemakers are increasingly being replaced by dual-chamber systems, it is crucial to understand single-chamber timing cycles before moving on to dual-chamber timing cycles, probably the most complicated subject in implantable devices. Although timing cycles may seem complex, the basics of its pacing are actually very simple. A pacemaker's primary role is to replace the beat that is missing to maintain appropriate cardiac output. Therefore, if the device sees or senses the event that it is looking for, it inhibits. If it does not see the event it is looking for, it paces and captures. Even the world's most sophisticated pacemaker can only sense and pace. If the clinician can "think" like the pacemaker, he or she will know how the pacemaker will behave.

Further reading

Bernstein AD, Irwin ME, Parsonnet V *et al.* Report of the NASPE Policy Conference on antibradycardia pacemaker follow-up: effectiveness, needs, and resources. NASPE. *PACE* 1994; **17** (11 Part 1): 1714–29.

Fraser JD, Gillis AM, Irwin ME *et al.* Guidelines for pacemaker follow-up in Canada: a consensus statement of the Canadian Working Group on Cardiac Pacing. *Can J Cardiol* 2000; **16**: 355–63, 367–76.

Levine PA. *Guidelines to the Routine Evaluation, Programming, and Follow-Up of the Patient with an Implanted, Dual-Chamber, Rate-Modulated Pacing System.* Sylmar, CA: St Jude Medical, 2003.

Schwaab B, Frohlig G, Berg M *et al.* Five-year follow-up of a bipolar steroid-eluting ventricular pacing lead. *PACE* 1999; **22**: 1226–8.

The nuts and bolts of single-chamber pacing

- The pacing threshold is the minimum amount of energy required to consistently and reliably capture the heart.
- Functional non-capture occurs when the pacemaker spike falls into the heart's intrinsic refractory period. During this period, the heart is electrically incapable of responding to the pacemaker output.
- Another cause of non-capture can be an output pulse that does not have enough energy to depolarize the heart.
- The pacing threshold is unique to each person and is subject to change over the course of the day, with disease progression, drugs, and even posture. In other words, the pacing threshold is not a fixed value.
- The safety margin is the amount added to the pacing threshold for programming a pacemaker output to assure that the pacemaker will capture the heart, even if the pacing threshold changes.
- Pacemaker outputs are defined by voltage (pulse amplitude) and milliseconds (pulse width).
- It is more energy efficient to increase the voltage (pulse amplitude) to increase pacing output energy than to increase the pulse width. (Doubling the voltage can quadruple the energy, while doubling the duration only doubles the energy.)
- The sensing threshold is the minimum sensitivity setting that allows for reliable sensing in the pacemaker.
- Sensing is determined by the sensitivity setting. A high value in the sensitivity setting means the device is less sensitive; a low value makes the device more sensitive.
- Oversensing leads to underpacing. Undersensing leads to overpacing.
- Pacing is governed by timing cycles. The main ones are the "alert period" when the device actively looks for and will respond to sensed signals and the "refractory period" when the pacemaker will not respond to signals.
- The base rate or lower rate is programmed in pulses per minute but defines a base rate interval commonly known as the lower-rate interval. Setting the base rate to 60 ppm results in a 1000 ms lower-rate limit interval.
- The most common single-chamber pacing mode is VVI and its rate-responsive version VVIR. VVT and VOO are used more frequently for temporary diagnostic purposes. Atrial single-chamber pacemakers (AAI) are not common.

CHAPTER 10

Dual-chamber pacing

Dual-chamber timing cycles can be complicated, because dual-chamber pacing is much more than an atrial pacemaker and a ventricular pacemaker working together. The main benefit of dual-chamber pacing is AV synchrony, the properly timed and coordinated activity of the atria in relationship to the ventricles. The healthy heart provides 1:1 AV synchrony, meaning that every atrial contraction results in a corresponding ventricular contraction. When AV synchrony prevails, patients have good hemodynamics and an efficiently pumping heart. When AV synchrony is disrupted or eliminated, patients can develop a host of symptoms.

Dual-chamber pacemakers provide AV synchrony by coordinating atrial activity with ventricular activity in such a way that 1:1 AV synchrony is encouraged, if not totally maintained. To accomplish this, the pacemaker has certain preset timing intervals on the atrial channel and other timing intervals on the ventricular channel. These cycles can sometimes "interlock" in that an event on the atrial channel may be the trigger for a ventricular timing cycle and vice versa.

There are really only three main timing cycles for the atrial channel and three for the ventricular channel (Table 10.1). (These main timing cycles may consist of several parts.) Both channels have one timing cycle in common: the alert period. The alert timing cycle is the regularly recurring interval of time during which the pacemaker can sense and respond to incoming signals. No pacemaker – even a single-chamber system – is alert all of the time. A constantly alert pacemaker would pick up and perhaps respond to inappropriate signals. To encourage the pacemaker to detect proper signals, the device is alert only at certain specific moments when atrial signals (the atrial alert period) or ventricular signals (the ventricular alert period) are likely to occur.

The atrial alert period

The atrial alert period refers to the specific time period on the atrial channel when the pacemaker seeks and can respond to atrial signals (Fig. 10.1).

If a P wave occurs during the atrial alert period, it immediately terminates the atrial alert period, i.e. the alert period ends as soon as it has sensed what it has been looking for.

Alert periods on both channels are precisely timed intervals. If the atrial alert period should expire or time out before it can sense a P wave, then the pacemaker will deliver an atrial output pulse.

The atrial alert period can only terminate if intrinsic activity is sensed, that is, if a P wave is detected, or if the alert period times out and an atrial output pulse is delivered.

The AV delay

In the healthy heart, the atria contract, then there is a pause, which is followed by a ventricular contraction. This pause, which occurs when electrical signals are temporarily and briefly delayed at the AV node, is what gives the healthy heart the proper AV synchrony it needs to pump efficiently. This pause between atrial systole and ventricular systole allows

Table 10.1 Timing cycles

Atrial channel	Ventricular channel
Atrial alert period	Ventricular alert period
AV delay or PV delay	Ventricular blanking period/ crosstalk detection window
PVARP	Ventricular refractory period

DDD Timing

AV = AV Delay

PVARP = Post Ventricular Atrial Refractory Period

*VBP = Ventricular Blanking Period

TARP = Total Atrial Refractory Period

VRP = Ventricular Refractory Period

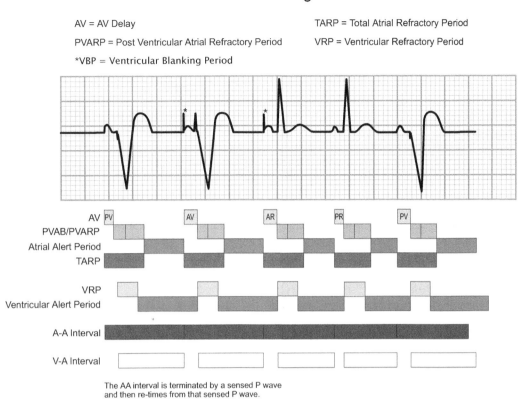

The AA interval is terminated by a sensed P wave
and then re-times from that sensed P wave.

Fig. 10.1 How the timing cycles of dual-chamber pacemakers build on each other and interact. The first illustration depicts the atrial alert period, the timing cycle during which the atrial channel can sense and respond to atrial activity.

for the atrial contribution to ventricular filling. Dual-chamber pacemakers mimic the healthy human heart by incorporating a timing cycle that creates this "rest" or pause between an atrial event (either paced or sensed) and the corresponding ventricular event.

The AV delay starts with an atrial event and allows a precisely timed interval to occur during which the pacemaker looks for ventricular activity. The AV delay is sometimes called the "paced AV delay" or the "sensed AV delay" depending on whether the atrial event that just occurred was sensed (i.e. intrinsic) or paced. While the AV delay is usually considered an atrial timing cycle (because an atrial event initiates it), it seeks activity on the ventricular channel to terminate it. The paced AV interval may also be

called the AP–VP interval, while the sensed AV interval may be called the AS–VP interval.

For most patients, the paced AV delay should be longer than the sensed AV delay. This owes not to any functional difference in the timing cycles but rather in how the pacemaker is able to initiate a timing cycle. A paced AV delay is launched with the delivery of an atrial output pulse. A sensed AV delay, on the other hand, actually commences and nearly peaks before the pacemaker is able to see and count it. As such, there is a short gap of time (known as "latency") by which the sensed AV delay timing cycle gets delayed. Most modern pacemakers allow independent programming of the sensed and paced AV delays and generally recommend that the sensed AV delay be *c.* 20 ms shorter than the paced AV delay.

The sensed AV delay (which corresponds to the "sensed AV interval") terminates when a ventricular event occurs. If an intrinsic ventricular event occurs at the right time, then the sensed AV delay terminates with an R wave. If the sensed AV delay times out before any intrinsic activity is sensed in the ventricle, then the pacemaker will deliver a ventricular output pulse.

PVARP

Just as important as the alert timing cycles, when the pacemaker looks for intrinsic activity, are periods of time when the pacemaker does not respond to any incoming signals. During these so-called refractory periods, the pacemaker will ignore incoming signals (or, in some cases, not even see them). The purpose of refractory periods is to prevent the pacemaker from responding to inappropriate signals. For instance, the atrial channel might "see" a ventricular paced event and detect electrical energy, which it could inappropriately interpret as a P wave. While clinicians have the benefit of viewing events on a rhythm strip, the pacemaker sees only electrical signals. To the pacemaker's sense amplifiers, a P wave "looks" exactly like an R wave or a T wave.

One crucial timing cycle in the dual-chamber pacemaker is known as PVARP, which stands for post-ventricular atrial refractory period. Its name describes its function exactly. The PVARP makes the atrial channel refractory after any ventricular activity. This means that the atrial channel will be immune from any major electrical signals which might reach the pacing lead following a ventricular contraction. (Since the ventricles are very large, they are very "loud" in terms of generating signals.) The purpose of the PVARP is to make sure the atrial channel does not sense any signals inappropriately (which would cause it to count an atrial event and launch a sensed AV delay). A ventricular event launches the PVARP, which makes the atrial channel refractory to incoming signals.

The PVARP is sometimes described in pacemaker manuals as consisting of subsets of other timing cycles. The post-ventricular atrial blanking period or PVAB may precede the PVARP, and the two together (PVAB + PVARP) form the refractory period on the atrial channel. Technically, the PVAB refers to a timing cycle in which the atrial channel is absolutely blind to incoming signals; it cannot see them. The PVARP refers to a timing cycle in which the atrial channel will not respond to any incoming signals, *although it can still see them*. The two timing cycles together, PVAB and PVARP, function as an atrial refractory period, a timing cycle during which the atrial channel is unresponsive to incoming signals.

The reason for differentiating a PVAB and a PVARP involves some advanced pacemaker features, such as mode switching, which are covered in more depth in a later chapter. PVARP makes the atrial channel unresponsive, but by seeing and counting atrial activity, it can help assess whether high-rate atrial activity is occurring.

The PVARP is a timing cycle that must time out every single time. When it expires, the next atrial alert period begins.

Thus, the sequence on the atrial channel is:
- atrial alert
- an atrial event (P wave or atrial output pulse)
- sensed or paced AV delay
- PVARP.

This cycle repeats continuously. It can vary, depending on whether the events are paced or intrinsic, but it always involves an alert period, an atrial event, an AV delay, and PVARP.

The ventricular refractory period

The ventricular refractory period is triggered by any ventricular activity on the ventricular channel, either sensed or paced. A ventricular event launches a ventricular refractory period, during which the pacemaker will not respond to any incoming signals. Just like on the atrial channel, this refractory period is actually composed of two parts: the first part is absolute (during which the ventricular channel is blind to incoming signals) and the second part is relative (the ventricular channel can see activity, but will not respond to it). The ventricular refractory period prevents the ventricular channel from inappropriately responding to incoming signals by counting it as a ventricular event.

The PVARP must time out before the next atrial alert period can begin. Any type of ventricular event launches a ventricular refractory period on the ventricular channel at the same time as it launches the PVARP on the atrial channel.

The ventricular blanking period and crosstalk detection window

Depending on how pacing leads are placed, the patient's anatomy, and the size of the output pulse, it is possible for an atrial output pulse to be picked up by the ventricular pacing electrode and "sensed" as some sort of ventricular activity. This phenomenon was observed on older pacemakers, which had no particular timing cycle mechanisms to prevent this from happening. Dubbed "crosstalk" because it involves the atrial channel inappropriately giving signals to the ventricular channel, it could interfere with normal dual-chamber pacemaker function. Modern pacemakers offer a ventricular blanking period and a crosstalk detection window to guard against the phenomenon.

The danger of crosstalk is crosstalk inhibition, in which the atrial output pulse is sensed on the ventricular channel, leading to inhibition of ventricular pacing.

The ventricular blanking period (VBP) and crosstalk detection window are two timing cycles which occur one immediately after the other. During the VBP, the ventricular channel is totally blind to incoming signals. During the crosstalk detection window, the ventricular channel may still pick up signals, but it will not respond to them.

These timing cycles occur *only* after a paced atrial event. They do not occur after intrinsic atrial activity, because native atrial contractions do not create crosstalk.

The ventricular alert period

Just like the atrial channel, the ventricular channel has a relatively long time interval during which it can detect and respond to ventricular activity. This timing cycle occurs when the ventricular refractory period times out.

The atrial escape interval

The atrial escape interval (AEI) may be easier to remember by its other name: the V-to-A interval. The AEI is not a consistent occurrence on a dual-chamber rhythm strip. It only occurs when an atrial paced event is followed by a ventricular event (either paced or sensed). The AEI or V-to-A interval represents the length of time the pacemaker will wait before an atrial output pulse is delivered. (Note that pacemakers may be based on ventricular timing or atrial timing; the AEI or V-to-A interval applies only to devices with ventricular timing.)

To calculate the AEI or V-to-A interval, start with the programmed rate and subtract the programmed paced AV delay. For example, if the pacemaker is programmed to a base rate of 60 ppm and a paced AV delay of 200 ms, first convert the base rate to the base interval (60 ppm = 1000 ms) and subtract (1000 − 200) to arrive at 800 ms. This is the AEI for that pacemaker, and the tracings from that device should show the timing between any ventricular event followed by a paced atrial event to be 800 ms.

For pacemakers with ventricular-based timing, the AEI or V-to-A interval remains constant. Other timing cycles may be adjusted as needed, but this one remains steady.

For pacemakers with atrial-based timing, the constant interval is the A-to-A interval, the time period between one atrial event (either sensed or paced) and the next paced atrial event (providing there are no intervening sensed atrial events).

Pacemakers are manufactured based on atrial timing or ventricular timing; it is not programmable. The issue of ventricular versus atrial timing cycles only occurs when analyzing ECGs. Either the AEI will be constant (pacing interval-AV delay) or the A-to-A interval will be constant (equal to pacing interval).

Rate-responsive AV delay

Despite the name, "rate-responsive AV delay" has more to do with normal DDD timing cycles than rate-responsive or sensor-driven pacing. The theory behind rate-responsive AV delay (RRAVD) is to mimic the healthy heart. In a normal heart, as the rate increases, the length of time shortens that the electrical signal is delayed at the AV node. The RRAVD (which may be a sensed or paced AV delay) allows the delay after the paced or sensed atrial event to be shortened appropriately in response to faster rates. This may occur during sensor-driven rate-responsive pacing, but it may also occur when the patient's own sinus node drives up the rate. The pacemaker automatically shortens the sensed or paced AV delay as the rate increases.

Fortunately for the clinician, the RRAVD does not require rigorous calculations. In most pacemakers, it can be activated and then allowed to use its own built-in algorithms to automatically adjust the delay timing cycle in relationship to the rate. In other words, it is a parameter that can be programmed ON or OFF, as needed. Some devices allow the RRAVD to be programmed to high, medium or low, in which high represents the most aggressive shortening of the delay timing cycle. The medium setting is generally designed to be the most universally applicable.

PVARP and the ventricular refractory period (VREF) are other timing cycles that are potentially impacted by higher rates. In very advanced pacemakers, it is possible to program a rate-responsive PVARP/VREF setting. In this instance, as the rate goes up, the device automatically shortens the PVARP and the VREF appropriately. Again, this is programmed by selecting high, medium or low settings, in which high represents the most aggressive shortening. This setting reduces both PVARP and the VREF concurrently, but in such a way that it attempts to maintain a 25 ms "spread" between the PVARP and the VREF, i.e. it tries to keep the PVARP 25 ms longer than the VREF.

For active patients with good sinus response or a rate-responsive pacemaker, it is often appropriate to allow for a relatively high sensor-driven or intrinsic rate. For this reason, some pacemakers allow the clinician to define the shortest PVARP/VREF setting in advance. The shortest PVARP/VREF is a boundary setting, defining the lowest values allowed for these two parameters. Even if otherwise indicated by the rate-responsive PVARP/VREF parameter, the device will not go below the programmed shortest PVARP/VREF settings. The nominal setting for shortest PVARP/VREF is 200 ms.

There are a couple of advantages to using these so-called "rate-responsive" settings. For patients who frequently experience higher rate activity (whether paced or sensed), these special parameters can help the pacemaker function more appropriately. By decreasing the refractory periods (PVARP and VREF) during periods of higher rate pacing, the pacemaker allows for more sensing of intrinsic events – events that might have otherwise fallen into the longer refractory period and been missed by the pacemaker. More sensing reduces the chance of competitive pacing, which is defined as pacing on top of intrinsic activity.

The four states of DDD pacing

Another way of thinking about dual-chamber pacing is to get down to the basics. A pacemaker can only do two things: sense or pace. Combine these activities for each channel, and there are only four combinations of activities that can occur, which have come to be known as the "four states of DDD pacing" (Table 10.2, Fig. 10.2).

As shorthand, an atrial paced event is AP, and a ventricular paced event is VP. An atrial sensed event is AS and a ventricular sensed event is VS. The four states of DDD pacing are AP–VP, AP–VS, AS–VP, and AS–VS.

Atrial tracking

The pacing state AS–VP is sometimes known as "atrial tracking," because the ventricular pacing rate

Table 10.2 The four states of DDD pacing

State	What it means
AV	An atrial paced event followed by a ventricular paced event
AR	An atrial paced event followed by a ventricular sensed event
PV	An atrial sensed event followed by a ventricular paced event
PR	An atrial sensed event followed by a ventricular sensed event

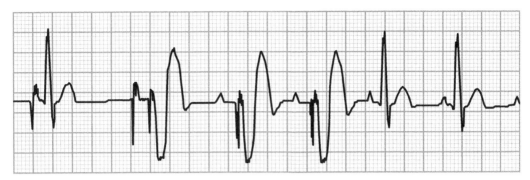

Fig. 10.2 The four states of DDD pacing are AP–VS, AP–VP, AS–VP, and AS–VS. The unpaced, healthy human heart beats in only one state: AS–VS.

follows or tracks to the atrial activity. This type of pacing works quite well, as long as the atrial rate remains within normal limits appropriate to the activity level. If the atria start to beat very quickly, the pacemaker will pace the ventricles rapidly in response. In the case of an atrial tachyarrhythmia, this can become uncomfortable or even dangerous for the patient. It is quite possible for a patient with atrial tracking to experience paced ventricular rates of 100 or 120 ppm in response to a high atrial rate.

For this reason, pacemakers offer an upper rate limit or "speed limit," sometimes known as the maximum tracking rate (or MTR, also known as max track). The MTR defines the upper rate limit, which is the highest rate at which the ventricles can be paced in response to atrial activity. The MTR works by imposing an upper rate limit timing cycle that overrides the sensed AV delay, forcing the pacemaker to postpone a ventricular output pulse until the upper rate limit interval times out (even if the sensed AV delay would have allowed one sooner).

Upper rate behavior

The goal of DDD pacing is to put in whatever beat is missing. But what if the beat that occurs is not appropriate? For example, what will the dual-chamber device do when the atrial rate accelerates? The timing cycles of a DDD pacemaker allow it to track up to and including the upper rate limit (or speed limit) or MTR. Some patients, however, will have the ability to increase their sinus and or atrial rates above this speed limit.

The DDD pacemaker has certain responses to these events that are called "upper rate behavior." Intrinsic atrial signals that fall into refractory periods will be tracked. Therefore, the behavior exhibited will be more atrial events than ventricular paced events. If an atrial event falls outside of the PVARP and initiates a sensed AV delay and pacing at the end of this delay would violate the upper tracking limit, the device will postpone the ventricular output until the upper rate limit interval has timed out.

This extension of the sensed AV interval waiting for the MTR to time out is called a Wenckebach response from the pacemaker. It mimics physiological Wenckebach behavior, in that if the atrial rate remains elevated, the sensed AV interval will get longer and longer until eventually a P wave falls inside the PVARP and is ignored by the device. On the surface ECG, the sensed AV interval gets progressively longer until a P wave is dropped. The following sensed AV interval shortens again and the process starts again.

When programming the pacing parameters in the DDD pacemaker, there is a refractory period that occurs as a result of the chosen parameters. It is called the total atrial refractory period or TARP. TARP is actually a combination of the PVARP plus the sensed AV delay. If and when the atrial rate accelerates faster than the TARP, multiblock occurs.

Let us take an example of a patient with a DDD pacemaker programmed to a base rate of 60 ppm, which translates into a pacing interval of 1000 ms. This patient has a paced AV delay programmed to 175 ms, a sensed AV delay set at 150 ms, an MTR of

120 ppm (500 ms), and a PVARP of 350 ms. These are fairly common settings. In this example, the patient has complete heart block so there is no conduction from the atria to the ventricles.

If this patient experienced atrial rates above 60 bpm, the device would track the atrium. That is, the pacemaker would try to "fill in the missing beat" so that every atrial event was followed by a (paced) ventricular beat.

The TARP value for this patient would be 500 ms (PVARP + sensed AV delay or 350 ms + 150 ms), which translates to a rate of 120 bpm Should the patient's intrinsic atrial rate exceed 120 bpm, multiblock will occur (Fig.10.3). This occurs because if atrial events are occurring faster than TARP, every other one will fall into the TARP and be missed by the pacemaker.

In short, when the patient's atrial rate goes over 120 bpm, the device will only track every other P wave, effectively cutting the ventricular rate in half.

This may be a great pacemaker response, but it is not necessarily the best hemodynamic response for the patient.

Staying with our example, this patient might be more comfortable and better served with a Wenckebach response. All of the settings stay the same (base rate 60 ppm, paced AV delay 175 ms, sensed AV delay 150 ms, MTR 120 ppm) except the PVARP. Instead of a PVARP value of 350 ms, let us reduce it to 250 ms.

The TARP value for this patient is 400 ms (PVARP + sensed AV delay or 250 + 150 ms). The 400 ms can be converted to a rate of 150 bpm. Now the intrinsic atrial rate has to exceed 150 bpm before multiblock will occur. Thus, reprogramming the PVARP to a shorter value has effectively changed the TARP value and permitted pacemaker Wenckebach to occur (Fig. 10.4). Another way of looking at this situation is that *shortening the PVARP value delays the onset of multiblock.*

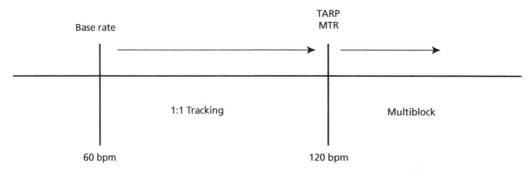

Fig. 10.3 As long as the intrinsic atrial rate is below the MTR and TARP value of 120 bpm, 1:1 AV synchrony occurs. If the intrinsic atrial rate should increase over 120 bpm, multiblock occurs.

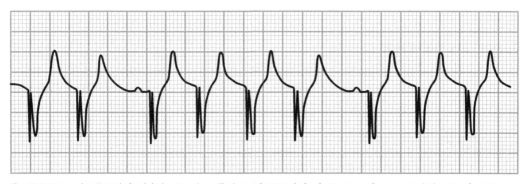

Fig. 10.4 Pacemaker Wenckebach behavior, also called pseudo-Wenckebach, is a type of upper rate behavior of a DDD pacemaker in response to rapid intrinsic atrial rates. The most common pattern for pacemaker Wenckebach is a 5:4 or 4:3 ratio.

When programming such settings, remember that the most optimal physiological response to an increasing intrinsic atrial rate is 1:1 tracking, i.e. matching every paced atrial event to a ventricular response. But as atrial rates accelerate, this might not be appropriate. By carefully programming the pacemaker, the clinician can allow for a Wenckebach response, giving the patient pacing support that is more physiological than multiblock.

Pacemaker multiblock occurs when every second or third (or other) atrial event is properly sensed. For example, 2:1 multiblock means two atrial events have to occur in order for one to be sensed, or, put another way, there are two atrial events for every resultant ventricular event (Fig. 10.5). The onset of multiblock occurs when the ventricular paced rate is suddenly cut in half, which many patients understandably find quite uncomfortable.

Pacemaker Wenckebach (the preferred upper rate behavior in the presence of high atrial rates) occurs only as long as the intrinsic atrial rate is greater than the MTR but less than TARP. For example, if the sensed AV delay is 200 ms and the PVARP is 200 ms, then TARP is 400 ms (200 + 200). If the interval of the patient's intrinsic atrial rate interval was less than 400 ms, then normal atrial tracking or possibly pacemaker Wenckebach would occur. This may be better understood by converting the intrinsic atrial rate interval of 400 ms to the corresponding rate of 150 bpm (Fig. 10.6).

On the other hand, if the patient's intrinsic atrial rate exceeds TARP, then the stage is set for pacemaker multiblock to occur. Many pacemaker programmers will calculate on screen the native atrial rate at which multiblock will occur. (The formula is simple: pacemaker multiblock will occur when the atrial rate exceeds TARP and TARP is the PVARP + sensed AV delay.) Using the above example of a 400 ms TARP, this means that multiblock will occur whenever the patient's intrinsic atrial rate is 150 bpm or greater.

From a hemodynamic standpoint, one-to-one tracking (1:1) is the most physiological response. At some high rates, however, 1:1 tracking would not be

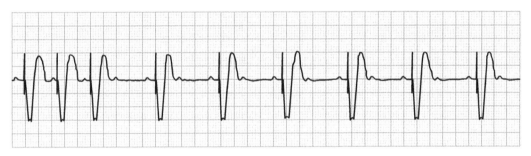

Fig. 10.5 Upper rate behavior may appear like 2:1 block on the ECG.

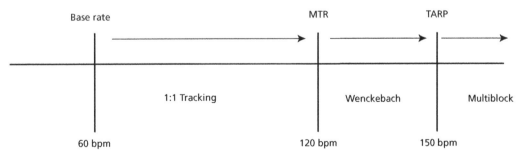

Fig. 10.6 As long as the patient's intrinsic atrial rate is below the MTR of 120 bpm, 1:1 AV synchrony occurs. By shortening the PVARP, a "window" is created between MTR and TARP. If the patient's atrial rate is faster than the MTR but slower than the rate associated with TARP, pacemaker Wenckebach will occur. Multiblock can still occur, but now only at rates above 150 bpm.

appropriate. Therefore, the device needs to be programmed to force some form of upper rate behavior. There are several key points to keep in mind:

- raise the MTR (if appropriate)
- program the sensed AV delay so it is shorter than the paced AV delay (TARP is actually PVARP + sensed AV delay)
- program RRAVD, that is, a sensed AV delay which will shorten automatically when the atrial rate increases.

The goal is to delay multiblock as long as possible, which is accomplished by creating Wenckebach behavior between the MTR and the TARP.

Modern pacemakers offer a very useful special feature known as mode switching, which can help avoid problems of upper rate behavior by basically switching off the atrial channel during periods of high atrial rate activity. For older pacemakers or those without mode switch algorithms, an understanding of upper rate behavior is essential to manage atrial tachycardias. These and other special features are treated in depth in a later chapter.

Dual-chamber modes

To understand the main timing cycles of dual-chamber pacing by mode, the following figures are good shorthand. By far, the most common dual-chamber mode for pacemakers is DDD (or the rate-modulated version of DDDR) (Fig. 10.7). This mode paces and senses both atrium and ventricle and it tracks the atrium.

The DDI or DDIR mode paces and senses in both chambers but does not track the atrium. For patients in the DDI mode, a high atrial rate will not cause a corresponding increase in ventricular paced response (Fig. 10.8).

DVI mode pacing is not a common programming choice, but it may be useful for some relatively rare cases, such as silent atria where dual-chamber pacing is required but atrial sensing is not desired (Fig. 10.9). In this mode, the pacemaker will pace both atrium and ventricle, but it only senses in the ventricle.

The DOO mode is asynchronous, meaning there is no attempt to time or synchronize the paced activity to intrinsic rhythms (Fig. 10.10). In this mode,

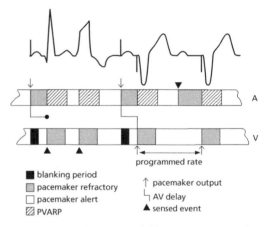

Fig. 10.8 DDI mode may be useful for patients with atrial tachyarrhythmias.

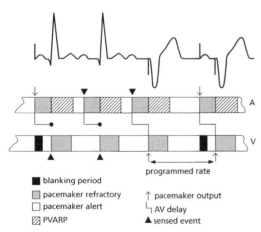

Fig. 10.7 The four states of dual-chamber pacing in the DDD mode.

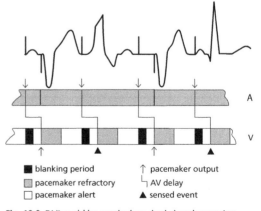

Fig. 10.9 DVI could be used when dual-chamber pacing is required but atrial sensing is not desired, such as in a patient with silent atria.

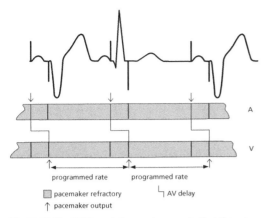

Fig. 10.10 The DOO mode is asynchronous in that there is no sensing and no attempt to synchronize paced events with intrinsic activity.

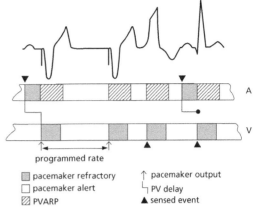

Fig. 10.11 VDD pacing requires functioning atria and AV block. The pacemaker may require only one lead, a "single-pass" lead which fixates in the ventricle and can sense the atrium through the blood pool with a floating atrial electrode.

both the atrium and the ventricle are paced, but there is no sensing at all. Consequently, the pacemaker does not respond or synchronize to intrinsic activity. DOO is contraindicated in the case of a competing intrinsic rhythm. It is rarely used except in cases when there is a need for dual-chamber pacing in the presence of significant interference, such as electromagnetic interference or electromyogenic (muscle) noise. Since interference can inhibit or trigger a pacemaker with sensing capabilities, the DOO mode provides pacing in a pacemaker-dependent patient, even in the presence of overwhelming noise.

The VDD mode warrants special consideration as a dual-chamber mode option. VDD or its rate-modulated version VDDR can be programmed in most dual-chamber pacing systems. There are also dedicated VDD and VDDR pacemakers, which usually rely on a single-pass lead (one lead that can pace and sense in the ventricle and which has a floating electrode to sense in the atrium through the blood pool). These so-called single-pass pacemakers offer specific benefits as they require only one lead (less hardware, less surgical time, decreased expense). They are indicated only for patients with normal sinus function and AV block (Fig. 10.11). Atrial tachyarrhythmia or sick sinus syndrome is a contraindication for a VDD pacemaker.

The main limitation to VDD pacing systems occurs if the sinus should later become incompetent. Such a patient is left with only ventricular pacing options.

Ventricular versus atrial timing

In the early days of dual-chamber pacing, all devices used what is commonly called ventricular-based timing. After a sensed or paced ventricular event, the VA interval started, also known as the atrial escape interval or AEI. At the end of the AEI, if no atrial activity was sensed, the device would deliver an atrial output pulse. This VA interval was set by a fixed millisecond value, based on the programmed lower rate limit of the device and the programmed AV delay.

For example, if a pacemaker was programmed to a base rate of 60 ppm (1000 ms pacing interval) and a paced AV delay of 200 ms, the VA interval would be 800 ms (pacing interval minus the paced AV delay = VA interval or AEI).

In a ventricular-based system, AP–VP pacing always occurs at the programmed base rate.

If after atrial pacing, however, the patient conducted intrinsically across the AV node, the resulting sensed QRS complex would initiate the fixed VA interval. This would cause atrial pacing at rates *faster than the programmed base rate.* This can appear confusing on a paced ECG.

In the mid-1980s, pacemaker manufacturers decided to fix this timing quirk by changing to what is now called atrial-based timing. In atrial-based timing, it is an atrial event (sensed or paced) that starts the interval known as the AA interval. This interval is the same as the programmed base rate. An atrial event also starts the sensed or paced AV interval. Therefore, the next time the device paces in the atrium is determined by the last time the atrium depolarized. With atrial-based timing, this method keeps the pacemaker from ever pacing above the programmed based rate, regardless of the faster conduction time across the AV node (Fig. 10.12).

Atrial-based timing introduced a new quirk. If the device goes from tracking behavior with a shorter sensed AV delay into AP–VP pacing, the V–V interval, when measured, will appear to be paced one beat slower than the programmed base rate. In reality, the base rate has not been violated because it is driven by A–A timing.

Another unique behavior with atrial-based systems occurs in the presence of premature ventricular contractions (PVCs). In the presence of a PVC, most devices will temporarily switch to V–A timing. When the pacemaker senses a PVC during the alert period, it times out the calculated VA interval by using the base rate minus the programmed paced AV delay and delivers the next atrial output pulse at the end of that interval.

Most implanted devices today use atrial-based timing. The most important issue to the patient is that regardless of which type of timing is used, the patient should not know the difference because timing changes are very small and have little to no effect on cardiac output.

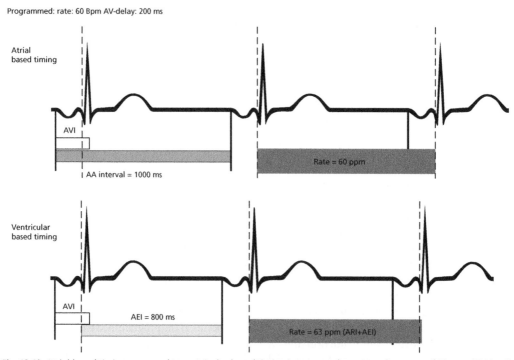

Fig. 10.12 Atrial-based timing compared to ventricular-based timing in a pacemaker set to a base rate of 60 ppm (1000 ms) with an AV delay of 200 ms. Ventricular-based systems could sometimes pace faster than the base rate, but atrial-based systems do not.

Further reading

Barold SS, Abe H, Nagatomo T. Paradoxical AV delay shortening of a pacemaker. *PACE* 2000; **23** (10 Part 1): 1527–31.

Barold SS, Fredman CS. Pure atrial-based lower-rate timing of dual-chamber pacemakers: implications for upper rate limitation. *PACE* 1995; **18** (3 Part 1): 391–400.

Bode F, Wiegand U, Katus HA *et al*. Inhibition of ventricular stimulation in patients with dual-chamber pacemakers and prolonged AV conduction. *PACE* 1999; **22**: 1425–31.

Eguia LE, Pinski SL, Haw J *et al*. Which is the optimal testing method for identifying an AV delay that allows intrinsic conduction? *PACE* 2000; **23** (11 Part 2): 1758–61.

Jutzy RV, Feenstra L, Pai R *et al*. Comparison of intrinsic versus paced ventricular function. *PACE* 1992; **15**: 1919–22.

Levine PA. *Guidelines to the Routine Evaluation, Programming and Follow-up of the Patient with an Implanted Dual-Chamber Rate-Modulated Pacing System.* Sylmar, CA: St Jude Medical, 2003.

Tse HF, Lau CP. The current status of single-lead dual-chamber sensing and pacing. *J Interv Card Electrophysiol* 1998; **2**: 255–67.

The nuts and bolts of dual-chamber pacemakers

- The goal of any dual-chamber pacemaker should be to provide to the greatest extent possible AV synchrony for the patient, i.e. a 1:1 relationship of atrial activity to ventricular activity.
- DDD pacemakers try to "fill in the beat" that is missing in the patient's own rhythm.
- A dual-chamber pacemaker has an atrial channel and a ventricular channel and timing cycles sometimes interlock, i.e. get initiated by an event on one channel and time out to cause an event on another channel.
- There are really only three main timing cycles for the atrial channel: the atrial alert period, the sensed or paced AV delay, and the PVARP.
- There are really only three main timing cycles for the ventricular channel: the ventricular alert period, the ventricular blanking period and crosstalk detection window, and the ventricular refractory period.
- The paced AV delay is the period between a paced atrial event and the next ventricular event (the ventricular channel is alert during the paced AV delay). The sensed AV delay is the period between a sensed atrial event and the next ventricular event (again, the ventricular channel is alert during the sensed AV delay).
- As a general rule, the sensed AV delay should be about 20 ms shorter than the paced AV delay because of a phenomenon known as latency. This means a P wave has partly occurred before the sensed AV timing cycle starts, whereas the paced AV delay starts as the atrial output pulse is delivered.
- PVARP is a refractory period on the atrial channel that occurs when a ventricular event occurs. Its purpose is to prevent the atrial channel from responding inappropriately to incoming signals from the ventricles.
- Ventricular activity triggers a short ventricular refractory period on the ventricular channel. The longest timing cycle on the ventricular channel is the alert period.
- When an atrial output pulse is delivered, a special ventricular timing cycle known as the ventricular blanking period (VBP) and crosstalk detection window result. These timing cycles prevent the ventricular channel from responding to any signals, such as they might obtain inappropriately from the atrial electrode.
- The danger of crosstalk is crosstalk inhibition, in which the atrial output pulse is sensed on the ventricular channel, leading to inhibition of ventricular pacing.
- Pacemakers may use ventricular-based or atrial-based timing cycles. This is not programmable. Most pacemakers today use atrial-based timing.
- In ventricular-based timing cycles, the atrial escape interval (AEI) or V-to-A interval remains constant. In an atrial-based timing cycle, the A-to-A interval remains constant. Other timing cycles may get adjusted to keep these constant.
- The AEI is defined as the time between any ventricular event (sensed or paced) and a following atrial paced event. To calculate the AEI, subtract the paced AV delay from the

Continued p. 88

Continued.

pacing interval. (For example, if the pacing rate is 60 ppm, the pacing interval would be 1000 ms. If the paced AV delay was programmed to 200 ms, then the AEI is 800 ms or 1000 − 200.)

- The A-to-A interval is the pacing interval. For example, if the pacing rate is 70 ppm, then the A-to-A interval is 857 ms.
- There are only four states in all DDD pacing: AP–VS, AP–VP, AS–VS, AS–VP.
- The maximum tracking rate (MTR) defines the fastest rate at which the ventricles can be paced in response to intrinsic atrial activity.
- Upper rate behavior occurs in pacemakers when there is high atrial rate activity in a dual-chamber tracking mode without mode switching.
- When a patient's intrinsic atrial rate exceeds the programmed MTR and TARP value, multiblock occurs.
- The onset of multiblock can be delayed by programming a shorter sensed AV delay. This shortens the TARP value (TARP = PVARP + sensed AV delay). When the intrinsic atrial rate is faster than the MTR but slower than TARP, pacemaker Wenckebach or pseudo-Wenckebach occurs.
- VDD pacemakers are often single-pass systems (requiring only one lead) and offer specific advantages but only for patients with reliable sinus activity and no atrial tachyarrhythmias.

CHAPTER 11

Basic paced ECG interpretation

Even clinicians who routinely evaluate ECGs can be challenged when viewing paced ECGs. Before presenting advanced material on special features and advanced timing cycles, it is important to understand the cornerstones of basic paced ECG interpretation. Like any part of pacemaker follow-up, paced ECG interpretation is best approached systematically. A mental checklist of items to evaluate on an ECG will not only allow clinicians to proceed more speedily through any follow-up session, but a system also helps assure that even obscure problems will not be overlooked.

In actual clinical practice, many paced ECGs are more complex than the ones presented in this chapter. But this chapter allows us to establish the basics of paced ECG interpretation, and, in the end, it is the basics that matter most.

Before evaluating these or any paced ECGs, it is important (if possible) to know the type of pacemaker and how it is programmed. In a routine pacemaker follow-up visit, this information should be available from the patient's chart and the telemetered data presented by the pacemaker. Knowing if the pacemaker is a single-chamber or dual-chamber system and how it is programmed allows the clinician to know what to expect.

The clinician should next look for pacemaker spikes, which indicate the delivery of an output pulse. Is there capture? Capture can be evaluated by determining whether a depolarization (AP or VP wave) occurs immediately after the pacemaker spike. This does not show that capture has occurred beyond a reasonable doubt, but it strongly suggests capture. Repeated occurrences of spikes and contractions make a solid case for capture. If the rhythm strip obtained does not have any pacemaker spikes, it is impossible to assess capture without doing further tests.

Next, sensing should be assessed. To evaluate sensing, an intrinsic event has to occur on the rhythm strip without a resulting pacemaker spike. If the pacemaker paces every cycle, it may not be possible to evaluate sensing from that particular strip.

Nowadays, the most accurate and reliable way to measure various intervals on the strip is to rely on annotations and markers. Intervals can, however, also be measured with calipers or by counting the grids on the ECG paper. (Each big square on the ECG grid counts as 200 ms. Each square is subdivided into five dots, with each dot representing 40 ms. Five big squares make up 1 s.)

There are some fundamental questions in interpreting basic paced ECGs.

1 What are the programmed settings of the pacemaker and are they consistent with what shows up in the rhythm strip?

2 Is pacing occurring at the proper rate?

3 Is there capture?

4 Is there sensing?

5 What is the underlying rhythm?

It is not always possible to find the answers to these five basic questions in every rhythm strip. Clinicians frequently have to dig a little during routine follow-up to make all of the necessary assessments on a pacing session. Nevertheless, these five basic questions can help any clinicians get a great deal of information out of even a very short basic rhythm strip.

Single-chamber pacemaker ECGs

There are pacing spikes that occur in the ventricular chamber in the first four complexes and in the last two complexes. The pacemaker offers annotation that spells out how many milliseconds elapse between that particular pacing spike and the next ventricular event (either VP or VS). Scanning the bottom of the strip in Fig. 11.1, it is clear that the first three complexes occur at precise 1000 ms intervals, which would translate to a pacing rate of 60 ppm.

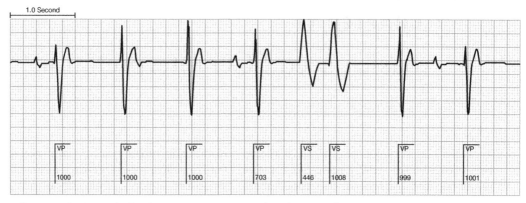

Fig. 11.1 The pacemaker is a single-chamber VVI system programmed to a base rate of 60 ppm.

The fourth complex starts with a paced ventricular event and ends with a sensed ventricular event (shown as VS) after just 703 ms. Since the R wave fell during the ventricular alert period, it was counted and resets the clock. Note that the next sensed ventricular event occurs after just 446 ms (which would translate to a pacing rate of about 134 ppm). However, it occurs during the ventricular alert timing cycle, so it also gets counted.

An interesting anomaly or unusual occurrence appears in the sixth complex where a particularly wide QRS complex is counted as a sensed ventricular event and the next ventricular paced event occurs 1008 ms later – this is longer than the programmed base rate. This slight increase over the programmed base rate (it amounts to pacing at 59.5 ppm instead of 60 ppm) occurs because the interval spans a sensed event to a paced event. When measuring rate on this sort of strip, it is important to measure V-to-V intervals. At times, however, slight variations (as in the final V-to-V interval) may occur.

To assess capture, it is important to find pacing spikes, which appear on this rhythm strip. Spikes on this strip occur almost on top of the ventricular event. Every spike is followed by a ventricular contraction. This is good evidence that capture is occurring.

To make a case for accurate sensing, it is necessary to find intrinsic ventricular events that get seen by the pacemaker. The presence of two VS annotations and two unpaced ventricular complexes which reset the timing cycles indicates that the pacemaker is seeing and properly responding to intrinsic ventricular activity. (Note that the intrinsic QRS complexes are

much wider than the paced ones; this is not uncommon.)

To assess the underlying rhythm, it is useful to look for atrial activity (it is intermittent) and how much pacing is going on. This patient is not getting the benefits of AV synchrony, but is receiving reliable ventricular pacing support. There is some native ventricular activity, which is properly sensed by the pacemaker.

Although the pacemaker spikes on the strip in Fig. 11.2 are small, it is clear that the pacemaker is delivering ventricular outputs. The paced rate cannot be accurately determined from this particular rhythm strip because there are no paced events followed immediately by a paced event (no V-to-V intervals) but the pacemaker spikes do appear at intervals of around 850 ms, which corresponds to a 70 ppm setting. Thus, the rate is probably right, but there is a much bigger problem going on.

The pacemaker spikes are not followed by a ventricular contraction. This means that the pacemaker is not capturing the ventricle. This strip illustrates very clearly the dangers of relying solely on annotations rather than looking at the strip itself. Whenever the pacemaker delivered a ventricular output pulse, the annotation noted a VP event, that is, a paced ventricular event. The strip, however, tells a different story. The output pulse was delivered, but there was no ventricular depolarization. The pacemaker "thinks" that ventricular pacing is happening, when, in effect, the device is not capturing the heart.

Ventricular sensing can be determined by looking for intrinsic ventricular activity and seeing if it is counted by the system and resetting the timers. This

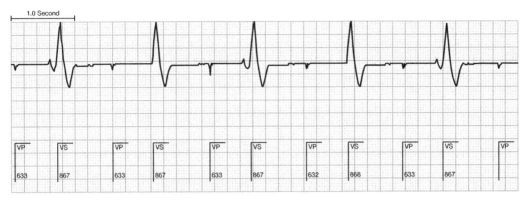

Fig. 11.2 The pacemaker is a VVI system set to a base rate of 70 ppm.

patient has a relatively stable series of intrinsic ventricular contractions marching through the strip. The pacemaker sees these events, annotates them as VS events and allows them to reset the timers. Thus, ventricular sensing is adequate.

The patient's underlying rhythm is actually fairly stable but slow (counting from one sensed ventricular event to the next results in roughly 1400 ms intervals which amount to a rate of about 43 bpm). Atrial activity is present but inconsistent. And the biggest issue on this strip is that the pacemaker is not capturing the heart!

Clinicians should avoid becoming overly dependent on annotations or markers on paced ECGs. In fact, the main value of such markers is confirmation rather than determination. The strip in Fig. 11.3 lacks the annotations, but it still contains all the information needed for a basic evaluation.

Although this is a paced ECG, there are no pacing spikes at all on this particular strip. Without even bothering to reach for the calipers, it is apparent that the heart rate is not stable. There is a long pause in the middle and even the rate between the seemingly stable complexes varies.

To determine capture, it is necessary to see a pacing spike followed by an immediate depolarization. There are no spikes on this strip, so capture cannot be determined. Further tests would be required to see if the system could capture.

Sensing is determined by evaluating whether the pacemaker sees intrinsic ventricular activity and uses it to reset the timer. Obviously, sensing must be going on in this strip, because the pacemaker is completely inhibited. But is sensing appropriate? Look at the long pause between the fourth and fifth pacing complex. An intrinsic ventricular event occurred; the pacemaker must have sensed it because it does not deliver a pacing spike. But the system was set to pace at 70 ppm, so after 857 ms (about four-and-a-half boxes on the grid), the device should

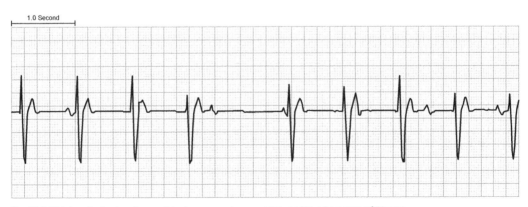

Fig. 11.3 This is a single-chamber ventricular pacemaker, programmed to a base rate of 70 ppm

have delivered a pacemaker spike to pace the ventricle. Instead, it did nothing. There is only one reason why the pacemaker would not deliver an output pulse: it was inhibited by something during the alert period. Yet looking at the rhythm strip, nothing was there to inhibit the device.

This is a case of "oversensing." The pacemaker sensed activity that was not actually present on the rhythm strip. An annotation might show up as a VS somewhere in the alert timing cycle. In actual fact, no intrinsic event occurred. A good way to remember this is that oversensing equals underpacing. The pacemaker did not pace where it needed to because it sensed something that was not there!

The rhythm strip in Fig. 11.4 shows a lot of ventricular activity. Look carefully, and there are some pacemaker spikes. They appear on this strip at the very tallest complexes. This sort of large pacemaker spike is usually made by a unipolar pacing system. There are seven pacemaker outputs on this strip, but there is a lot more ventricular activity than seven complexes.

There are a couple of places on the strip where a ventricular paced event is followed immediately by a ventricular paced event (a V-to-V interval). They appear in the first two and last two paced events on the strip as well as at two complexes in the middle of the strip. Measuring the intervals will reveal that the interval is about 850 ms, which is consistent with the 70 ppm setting.

To assess capture, it is necessary to see spikes followed by ventricular contractions. This occurs seven times on this strip, so there is reliable capture.

But what about sensing? To evaluate sensing, it is necessary to find intrinsic ventricular activity and see if the pacemaker recognized it and reset the timing cycles. There is no shortage of intrinsic ventricular activity on this strip. After the second paced

complex on this strip, a sensed ventricular event occurs. It is followed by another sensed ventricular event. Then, at the proper time, a paced complex comes in. This indicates good sensing.

Now look at the fourth tall QRS complex, indicating a pacemaker output pulse. Right after this paced event, there is an intrinsic ventricular event. This is followed closely by a tall paced QRS complex. In fact, the timing is such that the pacemaker output pulse was delivered within about 250 ms of the sensed ventricular event, i.e. much too quickly.

Why would the pacemaker pace the ventricle almost immediately after a sensed ventricular event? The only reason for this behavior is that the pacemaker did not see the sensed ventricular event. It missed it. It was timing the ventricular output based on the last paced ventricular event; it failed to recognize the intrinsic intervening event that should have reset the timing cycles.

This is known as ventricular "undersensing," which occurs when the pacemaker does not sense what it ought to sense. Another way to think of this is that undersensing leads to overpacing, i.e. pacing too frequently.

Dual-chamber pacemaker ECGs

Dual-chamber pacemaker ECGs involve more timing cycles and more pacemaker spikes, but can be approached in the same systematic fashion.

The device in Fig. 11.5 uses ventricular-based timing, so the AEI (atrial escape interval) at these settings would be 800 ms (1000 ms pacing interval minus the AV delay of 200 ms) or four grids on the ECG paper. The AEI is the time period between a paced ventricular event and the next paced atrial event. This can be seen at the very outset of the strip: the first paced ventricular event to the second paced

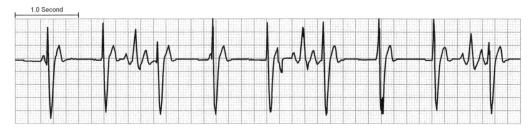

Fig. 11.4 This strip was taken from a pacemaker in VVI mode, set at a base rate of 70 ppm

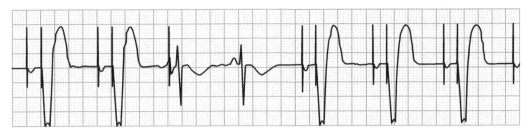

Fig. 11.5 This is a DDD pacemaker programmed to 60 ppm, with both paced and sensed AV delays set to 200 ms. The PVARP is 250 ms and the MTR is 120 ppm (500 ms).

atrial event measures 1000 ms. This pattern appears in several places on the strip. Thus, it *seems* that the pacemaker is pacing at the appropriate rate.

To assess capture, first consider the atrial channel. There are atrial pacing spikes and they are consistently followed by an atrial depolarization. This indicates proper atrial capture. On the third atrial beat, the pacemaker spike seems to be running right through the atrial depolarization. This is known as "fusion" and it occurs when a pacemaker spike is delivered as the chamber is already contracting. It could be thought of as a merger between a paced and sensed beat. Fusion is counted by the pacemaker as a paced event and it is not harmful to the heart.

On the ventricular channel, ventricular spikes are also consistently followed by ventricular depolarizations. Thus, there is appropriate capture in the ventricles. Both chambers are working well in this regard.

To evaluate sensing, intrinsic activity is needed. The fourth complex in the middle of this strip shows unpaced atrial and ventricular activity. The P wave (AS event) conducts to the ventricle. This event is seen by the pacemaker, in that it resets the timing cycles. Although there is only one unpaced complex, it is fair to say that there is apparent appropriate atrial and ventricular sensing. In this particular strip, the evidence gathered systematically supports the initial impression.

The AEI in Fig. 11.6 is 800 ms or four grids on the ECG paper and can be measured by counting from the first paced ventricular event (which is the first ventricular event on the strip) and the next paced atrial event (the second paced atrial event on the strip). The pacemaker rate *seems* to be correct.

To assess capture, it is necessary to find pacemaker spikes, which are present on this strip. In fact, every single atrial complex is preceded by an atrial pacing spike. This is evidence of atrial capture.

On the ventricular side, the ventricular pacing spikes are also followed by ventricular depolarizations. Ventricular capture is present. Note that there is some degree of fusion in the second paced ventricular complex.

For sensing, intrinsic events are required. Since every single atrial event on this rhythm strip is paced, it is impossible to evaluate atrial sensing from this strip alone. Further testing is required. Atrial sensing may be perfectly appropriate; there is just no evidence for it from this strip.

On the other hand, there are some unpaced ventricular complexes on the second half of the strip. It looks like the pacemaker paces the atrium, and the beat conducts down through the ventricles. Since

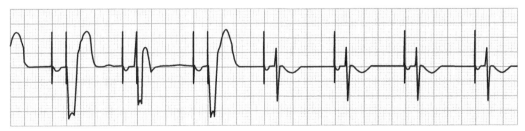

Fig. 11.6 This is a DDD system set at 60 ppm with a paced and sensed AV delay of 200 ms. The MTR is 120 ppm (500 ms) and the PVARP is 250 ms.

these ventricular events inhibit further ventricular pacing spikes, ventricular sensing is adequate.

Even without a neat AEI interval on the strip in Fig. 11.7, it is very apparent that pacing activity is occurring at a rapid rate. Although this is a dual-chamber strip, there are only pacemaker spikes for the ventricle. The atrium is beating on its own – and rapidly! In the very first complex, an intrinsic atrial event occurs followed by a ventricular pacing spike and ventricular depolarization. That complex alone gives good evidence of reliable atrial sensing and ventricular capture. The ventricles have just about depolarized when the next intrinsic atrial event occurs. This native atrial event prompts the pacemaker to deliver a ventricular output and pace the ventricle. It happens again with the third P wave: the atria are beating rapidly and the pacemaker is "tracking" the ventricle in response to the atrial activity. This means that the ventricular rate will be fairly rapid. In fact, if you measure the ventricular rate in these first complexes, it is over 115 ppm.

Over the course of even this short strip, the P wave appears earlier and earlier in the cycle. At first the P wave is right after the T wave, and then it moves up the T wave until finally it appears almost on top of the T wave as a little notch. This fifth P wave is the only one that is not followed by a ventricular output pulse. In fact, nothing happens after this fifth P wave except another P wave. The distance between this fifth P wave and the next P wave is about 480 ms (125 ppm) so the atria are beating fast. But the pacemaker misses this fifth P wave and does not come back with a ventricular response until the sixth P wave, effectively lowering the ventricular rate.

This is an example of "pacemaker multiblock," which has abruptly cut the ventricular paced rate in half. The mechanism behind pacemaker multiblock involves the post-ventricular atrial refractory period (PVARP). The PVARP is launched whenever there is a ventricular event; PVARP makes the atrial channel unresponsive to any incoming signals. In this particular strip, the PVARP is 250 ms. Every ventricular event launches a PVARP timing cycle on the atrial channel. The first few atrial events fell outside the PVARP, i.e. during the atrial alert period, so they were sensed. Since the atrial activity was sensed, the pacemaker responded to them by tracking the ventricle, i.e. pacing the ventricle in such a way as to encourage 1:1 AV synchrony.

But the fifth atrial event occurred during the PVARP. This means that although it occurred, the atrial channel on the pacemaker would not respond to it. The PVARP timed out and the first atrial event to occur during the atrial alert period was counted and used to time the next ventricular response.

Although it is not likely to be very comfortable for the patient, pacemaker multiblock is appropriate pacemaker upper-rate behavior. It is appropriate in that the pacemaker can be expected to do this whenever the intrinsic atrial rate exceeds the programmed MTR and the TARP (TARP = PVARP + PV delay). Pacemaker multiblock prevents the pacemaker from trying to track to a very quickly beating atrium.

While pacemaker multiblock may be "appropriate" pacing behavior at certain programmed settings, it may not be the most desirable option for the patient. One way to delay the onset of pacemaker multiblock is to shorten the PVARP value. Shortening the PVARP shortens the TARP value (remember: TARP = PVARP + sensed AV delay). In such cases, if the intrinsic atrial rate exceeded the MTR but did not exceed the TARP, then pacemaker Wenckebach would occur, at least until the point that the intrinsic atrial rate exceeded TARP. (See Chapter 10, Upper rate behavior.)

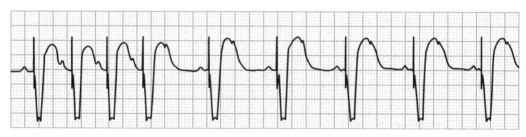

Fig. 11.7 This is a DDD pacemaker without mode switching, programmed to 60 ppm and an MTR of 120 ppm (500 ms). The paced and sensed AV delays are both 200 ms and the PVARP is 250 ms.

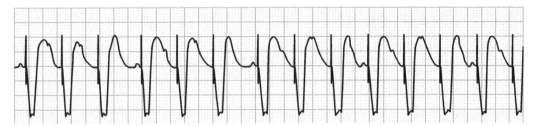

Fig. 11.8 This is a DDD device programmed to 60 ppm, MTR 120 ppm, with a paced and sensed AV delay of 150 ms and a PVARP value of 250 ms.

The final dual-chamber strip shown in Fig. 11.8 is another example of upper rate behavior in a dual-chamber pacemaker. Although the device is set to a base rate of 60 ppm, there is a lot of intrinsic atrial activity going on and the pacemaker is tracking the atria and causing the ventricles to be paced fairly rapidly. Every ventricular event starts the PVARP timing cycle, which makes the atrial channel unresponsive to incoming signals for 250 ms. That is why some of the intrinsic atrial events are followed closely by a ventricular pacing spike and ventricular depolarization, while other P waves seem to be "missed." If an intrinsic atrial event falls into the PVARP, it goes uncounted and there is no immediate ventricular pacing spike in response.

Studying this strip carefully, a pattern emerges. Sensed atrial events fall into the PVARP and get missed while a regular pattern of properly sensed atrial events results in a ventricular pacing output. This is an example of 3:2 "pacemaker Wenckebach" behavior. It is an appropriate upper rate response to a rapid intrinsic atrial rate. In fact, it mimics the way the healthy heart tries to equalize a rapid atrial rate.

Further reading

Dubin D. *Rapid Interpretation of EKG's*, 4th edn. Tampa, FL: Cover, 1993.

Ellenbogen KA. *Cardiac Pacing*, 2nd edn. Cambridge, MA: Blackwell, 1996.

Kenny T. *Nuts and Bolts of Paced ECG Interpretation*, 2nd edn. Oxford: Blackwell (in press).

Levine PA. *Guidelines to the Routine Evaluation, Programming and Follow-up of the Patient with an Implanted Dual-Chamber Rate-Modulated Pacing System*. Sylmar, CA: St Jude Medical, 2003.

The nuts and bolts of basic paced ECG interpretation

- Paced ECGS require some special interpretation skills beyond those used in the interpretation of standard ECGs. A systematic approach works best.
- There are five key questions to ask in basic ECG interpretation. What are pacemaker settings? What is the rate? Is there capture? Is there sensing? What is the underlying rhythm?
- To assess capture, it is necessary to see pacemaker spikes followed by depolarization. This is not always evident on every rhythm strip.
- To assess sensing, it is necessary to see intrinsic events that reset the timing cycles. This is not always evident on every rhythm strip.

- Annotations and markers can be useful on ECGs, but should be used for confirmation or assessment of what the pacemaker sees, rather than for ECG evaluation. For example, a pacemaker that is oversensing will "see" activity that is not present on the rhythm strip.
- Oversensing leads to underpacing, while undersensing leads to overpacing.
- Rapid intrinsic atrial activity can provoke "upper rate behavior" in dual-chamber pacemakers which mimics 2:1 block or Wenckebach. This is appropriate behavior for the pacemaker.

CHAPTER 12

Rate-responsive pacing

Rate-responsive (sometimes called rate-adaptive or rate-modulated) pacing developed in response to the clinical need to provide an adequate cardiac output for pacemaker patients. Few advanced pacemaker features have enjoyed such rapid and widespread acceptance as rate-responsive pacing. In fact, most modern pacemakers offer rate response as a nearly "standard" feature.

For frail, bedridden, or otherwise sedentary pacemaker patients, a single programmable base rate seemed to meet their needs. For patients who maintain even an ordinary lifestyle, which might include walking across a parking lot, mowing the lawn, carrying a sack of groceries and so on, the single programmable rate does not always meet their needs. Very active pacemaker patients, such as the ones who run marathons or climb mountains, clearly needed more than standard devices to accommodate their needs.

In hemodynamic terms, active people need more cardiac output than sedentary people. Cardiac output (CO) can be defined as the amount of blood (in liters) pumped through the heart in a minute. It is defined by the heart rate (HR) and the stroke volume (SV), which is the amount of blood (in liters) pumped through the heart in one single beat. The formula for cardiac output is simple:

$$CO = HR \times SV$$

To better appreciate this issue, consider the healthy heart. As metabolic demand increases (for example, during exercise) the sinoatrial (SA) node fires more rapidly, increasing the atrial rate which results in a faster ventricular rate. When metabolic demand decreases, the SA node fires more slowly, the atrial rate slows down, and the ventricular rate follows suit. This system does not work for patients with compromised sinus function, one of the main reasons for which pacemakers are prescribed. Add to that a better understanding of something known as chronotropic incompetence (the heart's inability

to pump in response to metabolic demand), and it is clear why so many pacemaker patients needed help in keeping heart rates appropriate for activity levels.

Pacemaker manufacturers sought ways to boost cardiac output by varying certain parameters. It was originally believed that increasing the paced ventricular rate would naturally elevate cardiac output. That turned out to be misleading, since raising the ventricular pacing rate for a patient at rest had a dampening effect on stroke volume resulting in a minimal or negligible improvement in cardiac output. In short, increasing the ventricular paced rate for a patient at rest did not significantly improve cardiac output (Fig. 12.1).

The missing link in the equation was physiological need, usually brought on by physical stress or exercise. If the body experienced metabolic demand, for instance brought on by physical exercise, then the higher paced ventricular rate *would increase* the

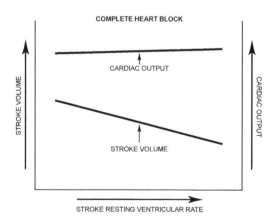

Fig. 12.1 When a person is at rest, increasing the ventricular rate has very little effect on cardiac output. As the resting ventricular rate goes up, stroke volume decreases, resulting in no significant net gain in cardiac output. For an increased rate to raise cardiac output, there must be a metabolic need.

---

cardiac output because stroke volume would remain constant or increase.

Thus, when it comes to accommodating pacemaker patients who are active, the preeminent parameter to look at is pacing rate.

For patients with a functional sinus node and chronotropic competence, an increase in activity causes the atria to beat faster. A properly programmed pacemaker will respond with rapid ventricular response to the intrinsic atrial rhythm. The increased pacing rate will drive up the cardiac output. The only brake on this type of system is the maximum tracking rate, which should be programmed with knowledge of the patient's activity level and anticipated "active" heart rates.

Chronotropic incompetence

Many pacemaker patients have (or are at risk of developing) a condition called chronotropic incompetence. Chronotropic incompetence means that the patient's heart rate does not increase rapidly enough, steeply enough, or sufficiently to meet the patient's metabolic demands (Fig. 12.2). Without

a rate-adaptive pacemaker, these are people whose natural heart rates would limit their activities.

Chronotropic incompetence is defined as an inadequate heart rate to meet metabolic need. It is typically assessed during exercise testing and may be evaluated as a heart rate that is < 120 bpm under any circumstances or a heart rate that cannot reach its maximum, calculated by subtracting the patient's age from 220 and then taking 90% of that value:

maximum HR < 90% of (220 – age) or

maximum HR < 120 bpm

Chronotropic incompetence is common in pacemaker patients and can be caused by age, heart disease, or certain medications. Pacemaker patients are often given a rate-responsive pacemaker even if they are not tested for chronotropic incompetence or have no signs of it, because chronotropic incompetence can develop suddenly in patients who did not have it previously.

To compensate for chronotropic incompetence and to provide increased pacing rates in the presence of physical activity, pacemakers were developed with sensors to help detect when there was a physical need for faster ventricular pacing. Rate re-

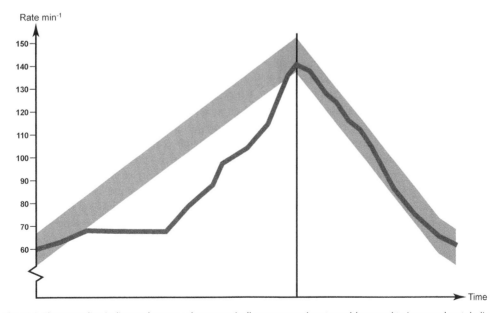

Fig. 12.2 The upper line indicates the way a chronotropically competent heart would respond to increased metabolic demand: it would beat progressively faster and, when metabolic demand ended, it would resume its resting rate. Chronotropic incompetence can take many forms; the lower line indicates a patient whose heart rate cannot ramp up quickly or evenly enough to meet metabolic demand. This is only one of any number of ways chronotropic incompetence could manifest itself.

sponse is probably the single most important factor in increasing cardiac output for active patients.

Sensor technology

Over the years, engineers and physicians have worked with a variety of variables and sensors to try to gauge increased patient need. The earliest sensors measured the pH value of venous blood. Others measured the temperature of the blood. These were all based on physiological changes during exercise that required an increase in metabolic rate.

It is generally held that blood temperature is a good indicator of physiologic demand. The reason blood-temperature-sensing pacemakers are not widespread is explained by two facts. The first is that sensing blood temperature requires a special lead and this specialized hardware poses special engineering challenges and limits the pacemaker to dedicated electrodes. The other problem with blood temperature as a variable is that it is slow. The physiological need of a person can go up sharply before blood-temperature-sensing electrodes can detect and respond to it.

Today, the most common sensors in use are activity sensors. These may be piezoelectrical crystals or accelerometers, both of which measure a physical variable and correlate it to activity. The piezoelectric sensor is sensitive to pressure waves, which would occur when the foot strikes the floor. Jogging creates more vibrations and would cause the piezoelectrical sensor to report higher activity levels than walking.

In 1985, Medtronic released the first rate-responsive single-chamber pacemaker. The Activitrax® pacemaker, as it was called, utilized a piezoelectric crystal bonded to the inside cover of the pacemaker. Its design made it sensitive to muscle vibration. When the patient's foot hit the floor, vibrations were created. This signal was transmitted to the pacemaker can and it bent the piezoelectric crystal. The amount of bend in the crystal determined the amount of rate acceleration given to the patient. The theory behind this was that more vibration meant more activity, more activity meant more demand, and more demand required rate acceleration. This was an effective sensor, but, like any sensor, it could be fooled. For example, imagine the footfall going downstairs versus going up. The rate might accelerate more going downstairs when physiologi-cally more acceleration is required going upstairs. The real advantage of the piezoelectric sensor was that it responded very quickly to activity. Most pacemaker patients exercise for short periods of time, so the rate acceleration they require needs to occur quickly.

A very reliable activity sensor is the accelerometer, which measures acceleration in one geometric plane. Accelerometers measure forward movement, such as would occur if a person started to run. The faster the person runs, the more forward motion the accelerometer would report.

These activity sensors are built into the pacemaker can and pick up signals in the form of vibrations (piezeoelectric sensor) or motion (accelerometer) and relay them to the pacemaker's circuitry for interpretation and response. If rate response is programmed on, detected activity will cause the paced rate to increase in order to increase cardiac output and keep the patient comfortable at higher levels of activity. Likewise, when the sensor detects less or no activity, the rate comes back down to the programmed base rate.

Accelerometers and vibration sensors are not as physiologic as sensors that detect blood temperature, but they do offer a couple of solid advantages which account for their widespread popularity. First, the sensor is built into the pulse generator (rather than being part of the lead). This allows an accelerometer-based rate-responsive pulse generator to be used with a wide range of leads – no special hardware is required. The other advantage of the accelerometer and the vibration (piezoelectric) sensor is speed. Accelerometers can quickly detect and respond to activity, causing the paced rate to increase almost immediately with motion.

Another approach to sensor technology has been the development of minute ventilation sensors. Minute ventilation is a sensor based on respiration (it measures how much lung movement occurs in a minute). Minute ventilation (MV) pacemakers require special leads that measure chest movements which correspond to breathing. If the MV sensor detects rapid breathing, the pacemaker responds with a higher rate.

Minute ventilation sensors require bipolar pacing leads. This may be a drawback when a unipolar pacemaker is in place. A physician cannot revise a unipolar pacing system with a minute ventilation device unless he or she is prepared to implant new pacing leads.

No pacemaker sensor yet devised is flawless. The two main issues with sensors are their degree of physiological response and response time. Accelerometers are responsive but not very physiologic. Minute ventilation is physiologic but not very fast. Temperature sensors are metabolic, but challenging to build and implement.

Furthermore, just about every sensor in use today can be "tricked" or at least misled. Piezoelectric sensors respond to vibrations and pressure. As such, they increase pacing rates much more walking downstairs (heavier footfall) than walking upstairs (lighter footfall), although walking upstairs is far more work to the body. Tapping the body around the implanted device can also cause the piezoelectric sensor to interpret these vibrations as activity, causing the pacing rate to go up.

Accelerometer sensors are not fooled by tapping or stairs, but as they measure forward motion, they can cause pacing rate increases when the patient is rocking in a rocking chair.

Minute ventilation sensors can increase the pacing rate inappropriately in the presence of big arm movements that the device interprets as respiration associated with chest movements.

Despite these drawbacks, rate response in modern pacemakers works well and reliably. Patients who experience inappropriate rate response should be cautioned against behaviors that might promote it (such as not tapping on the pacemaker or avoiding rocking chairs).

Programming rate-responsive pacemakers

Rate response involves a series of programmable parameters that start with the sensor itself. In some pacemakers, it is possible to program the sensor ON and OFF and even to a PASSIVE setting, which means that the sensor detects and stores signals but does not respond to them. (A passive setting is useful to see how the device would perform as a rate-responsive device before activating the rate-response function.)

Some sensors require the clinician to set a threshold value, which could be defined as the amount of activity necessary to initiate sensor activity. If the threshold is set too low, then even mild activities, such as getting up out of a chair or walking across the room could cause the sensor to take over the rate. On the other hand, if the sensor is too low, then the sensor cannot drive the rate unless the patient is moving vigorously. Threshold settings depend on the patient's lifestyle.

In addition, it is possible to program how rapidly rate response increases and decelerates the rate. These settings are usually described in terms of "slow," "medium" and "fast," with fast appropriate for the most active patients. This determines how steeply the sensor increases the rate in response to activity. In addition to response time (how quickly and how steeply the rate increase occurs), it may be possible to program the recovery time. This defines how quickly the rate goes back down to the base rate when the sensor determines that activity has decreased.

The slope of the rate is defined as the sensor-driven rate for a given activity level. For example, an aggressive slope would determine that the sensor-driven rates be fairly high for given activity levels. A mild slope would allow the sensor to drive the rate up only slightly for that same level of activity. Slope, like other parameters governing sensor behavior, should be programmed with an eye to the patient's lifestyle and activity level. The sensor settings for an elderly patient should not be as aggressive as sensor settings for an athlete. (Yes, some athletes have pacemakers.)

The maximum sensor rate is an important programmable setting intended to help control how fast the pacemaker will pace, even in the presence of strenuous physical activity. It is important to program a maximum sensor rate that accommodates the patient's lifestyle. Very active patients will need higher maximum sensor rates than sedentary ones.

Dual-sensor systems

Recent advances in cardiac pacing have developed a so-called dual-sensor system which attempts to balance out the strengths and weaknesses of various sensor systems by pairing the "best of both worlds." One dual-sensor system relies on a combination of minute ventilation sensing (physiologic benefit) and an activity sensor in the form of an accelerometer or piezoelectric crystal (rapid response). Another dual-sensor combination is blood temperature (physiologic) and activity (rapid response).

In a dual-sensor system, both sensors are active in the pacemaker but only one sensor controls the pacing rate at any given moment during sensor-driven pacing. The pacemaker's circuitry is able to receive, analyze, and sort through both incoming sensor signals and opt for the preferred signal at any given moment. In theory, the idea is that the more rapid sensor provides for the initial onset of rate response, allowing the more physiologic sensor to take over as it "comes up to speed."

Dual-sensor systems have not found widespread acceptance, although most clinicians with experience of such devices agree that they work well, possibly even somewhat better than the more popular single-sensor systems. The reason these devices are not in greater distribution is simple: they offer slightly improved rate response at a price of significantly more complicated programming and follow-up time. The slight improvement in sensor performance (which the patient may not even notice) is simply not worth the hours of extra time it can take to get both sensors properly programmed.

Rate-responsive settings

Advanced pacing systems have drastically simplified the way that rate response is programmed. Most programmable parameters associated with rate response allow the clinician to program how aggressive the rate response should be in response to sensor input. As a general rule of thumb, the more active the patient, the more rate-response settings can be aggressive. Sedentary, frail, or physically limited patients need the least aggressive forms of rate response.

During follow-up, sensor histograms should be downloaded and the amount of sensor-driven paced activity should be reviewed. The amount of sensor-driven activity and the rates to which the sensor drove the rates should be in keeping with the patient's age, abilities, and lifestyle. A wheelchair-bound patient who exhibits lots of high-rate sensor-driven pacing most likely needs the rate-responsive parameters adjusted.

Rate-responsive pacing review

Rate-responsive pacing is becoming so common, especially in the United States, that it is rare today to see new pacemaker systems implanted without a sensor. But not all sensors get activated. It is not unusual in clinical practice to see rate-adaptive systems functioning in non-rate-adaptive modes or to see sensors set at a PASSIVE rather than ON setting. There are a few reasons for this.

Some physicians prefer not to activate rate-adaptive settings at implant. It is often difficult for even an experienced pacemaker physician to anticipate how rate-modulated parameter settings will affect a new pacemaker patient. For that reason, some physicians will implant a pacemaker, activate the sensor to a PASSIVE setting, and then use histograms or other programmer settings to retrieve information on how the sensor would have driven the rate, had it been in control. This is usually done at one of the early follow-up settings. At this point, the doctor can see how high the sensor would have driven the rate and for how long. Depending on the patient's activity levels, lifestyle and the doctor's clinical judgment, the sensor settings can be fine-tuned at this point and then the sensor turned ON.

In the case of a very frail, bedridden, or sedentary patient, rate-modulated pacing may not be necessary to provide adequate pacing support. The sensor may be left PASSIVE or OFF in such cases. In other cases, the patient may not require a sensor for rate-adaptive pacing, but may need the sensor for such specialized features as the AF Suppression™ algorithm (which relies on an activity sensor) or the Auto Rest Rate. These and other specialized features will be the subject of the next chapter.

Further reading

Abrahamsen AM, Barvik S, Aarsland T et al. Rate-responsive cardiac pacing using a minute ventilation sensor. PACE 1993; 16: 1650–5.

Furman S, Hayes DL, Holmes DR Jr. A Practice of Cardiac Pacing, 3rd edn. Mount Kisco, NY: Futura, 1993.

Greenhut SE, Shreve EA, Lau CP. A comparative analysis of signal processing methods for motion-based rate-responsive pacing. PACE 1996; 19: 1230–47.

Katritisis D, Camm AJ. Chronotropic incompetence: a proposal for definition and diagnosis. Br Heart J 1993; 70 : 400–2.

Lukl J, Doupal V, Sovova E et al. Incidence and significance of chronotropic incompetence in patients with indication for primary pacemaker implantation or pacemaker replacement. PACE 1999; 22: 1284–91.

Rao G. Hemodynamic advantage of temperature-sensing rate-adaptive pacemakers. Int Surg 1993; 78: 262–5.

The nuts and bolts of rate response

- Rate modulated, rate responsive, rate adaptive all mean the same thing: the device contains a sensor to help adjust the rate in response to the patient's need.
- Most common sensors today are activity (mainly the accelerometer, some piezoelectric) and minute ventilation.
- When the sensor detects that the patient needs faster pacing support, the sensor drives the rate to the appropriate level.
- No sensor is perfect. Every sensor can be fooled. Some devices combine two sensors to take advantage of what is strong in each one. Typical dual-sensor devices combine an accelerometer and minute ventilation or an accelerometer and temperature.
- While dual-sensor systems are commercially available and the consensus is that they work well, many clinicians find them too "adjustment intensive" for the added benefit. This is often a matter of personal physician preference.
- Some pacemakers have automatically adjusting rate-responsive AV/PV delays, rate-responsive PVARP/VREF or similar settings to adjust timing cycles to higher rate, sensor-driven pacing.
- Most new devices in the US are rate-responsive pacemakers, but the sensor is sometimes turned OFF or to PASSIVE.
- Sensors are used not only for rate response, but also in certain special features, such as the AF Suppression™ algorithm or the Auto Rest Rate.

CHAPTER 13

Special features

The history of cardiac pacing has really been an ongoing progression of innovations. From the first pacemaker "cooked up" on the kitchen table of Swedish inventor Rune Elmqvist to devices currently on the drawing boards of pacing engineers today, progress can be measured in improvements, enhancements, and special features. Special features include a wide range of functions added to late-generation pacemakers to make them work better, last longer, improve therapy, or streamline follow-up and facilitate patient management.

Some of these "special features" have become so valuable to patients and clinicians that they have become almost "standard" functions for devices implanted today. For example, rate-responsive pacemakers were introduced as an innovative new approach to managing chronotropic incompetence. Today, most pacemakers implanted in the US offer rate response, even if the feature is not activated. Indeed, the demand for some of these special features can be seen in the fact that virtually all manufacturers offer them.

It can become a little confusing for novices in pacing therapy to confront the variety of features. Every manufacturer offers some variation on the features, both in terms of nomenclature and in functionality. Add to that the fact that these special features are constantly being improved, upgraded and enhanced, and even within one product family from one manufacturer, there can be subtle (and not-so-subtle) differences in how the same feature works.

For that reason, pacing clinicians – both those who deal with pacemaker patients frequently and those who follow pacemaker patients only occasionally – must obtain copies of the technical manuals (sometimes called physicians' manuals) for all devices. In most countries, the law requires all manufacturers to provide a printed manual in every single device package. Today in many regions, online or electronic manuals are permissible, but

manufacturers are glad (and often legally obligated) to provide clinicians with printed manuals upon request. Pacemaker sales representatives can also provide manuals and other valuable information on the devices they sell. Most manufacturers offer training programs, educational materials, and other opportunities to learn the specific functionalities of their products. The pacemaker representative should be considered the primary and best source for product-specific information.

For the purposes of this book, special features are described in broad, general terms whenever possible. In the world of device therapy, however, generics are not always possible. Thus, this book offers "big picture" descriptions and not necessarily the details for specific programming situations. For those details, it is best to supplement this book with pacemaker manuals and other training materials for the products most frequently encountered in clinical practice.

Special features are worth getting to know because they can optimize pacemaker therapy for patients, give clinicians more accurate diagnostic information, and make it easier for the physician to evaluate pacemaker behavior at follow-up. These special features can impact rhythm strips obtained during follow-up; when doing a systematic analysis of a paced ECG, note which (if any) of these special parameters are programmed.

Automatic mode switching

The concept of mode switching is very simple. If a dual-chamber pacemaker patient experiences a very high intrinsic atrial rate, the pacemaker will shut off the atrial channel until the rate gets back down to normal. Turning off the atrial channel means that the pacemaker won't try to track the ventricle to the high atrial rate, avoiding an uncomfortable (and potentially dangerous) rapid ventricular response.

When a DDD or DDDR pacemaker suddenly turns off its atrial channel in response to high atrial activity, this causes the device mode to change. In many modern pacemakers, the clinician can program how the mode should change. For example, the device might be programmed to change from DDDR to VVIR in the presence of high atrial rate activity.

To program mode switching, the clinician must establish a "trigger" or the intrinsic atrial rate that must be reached to initiate mode switching. Unfortunately, there is not a simple one-size-fits-all trigger value. In general:

- if the patient has an intact sinus node and is fairly active, set the trigger high to avoid causing the device to mode switch when the patient is exercising
- if the patient experiences a lot of high-rate atrial activity and is symptomatic at rapid ventricular response, set the mode switch lower to avoid rapid ventricular pacing
- patients with sick sinus syndrome may need mode switching if they ever experience high atrial rates.

Mode switching is programmed to become active when a certain number of events at the trigger rate occur within a certain time frame. This is usually formulated as a window (if x trigger-rate events occur in a window of y total events). At that point, the device changes mode, which means that the device no longer responds to atrial input.

The first devices with mode switching found that many patients experienced a rapid intrinsic atrial rate and a somewhat rapid ventricular response followed by a sudden drop in rate as mode switching kicked in. As can be seen in Fig. 13.1, the rate can lower significantly in just one beat. Some patients are particularly sensitive to such "bumps" in rate.

Therefore advanced mode switching algorithms allow for a so-called "Auto Mode Switch (AMS) base rate." This is a programmable rate that automatically goes into effect whenever a mode switch occurs. The AMS base rate should be programmed higher than the regular base rate but not uncomfortably high for the patient.

The duration of the mode switch is usually subject to programmable settings. Although the pacemaker does not respond to any atrial activity during the mode switch, it still "sees" and counts atrial events. When the atrial activity has gone back down below the trigger level for a programmable number of cycles, the device switches back to the originally programmed mode.

Mode switch episodes are counted by the device and are tracked. For diagnostic purposes, this information can be downloaded in the form of a report called a histogram. This histogram, usually in the form of a bar diagram, can help the clinician assess how much mode switching has been going on for the patient.

When examining a mode switch histogram, there are some key points to look for.

- A large amount of mode switch episodes indicates that the patient is either experiencing a lot of high rate atrial activity or that the device is programmed to a trigger that is too low for the patient.
- A patient who is experiencing a lot of high intrinsic atrial rate activity without mode switching suggests that the trigger is too high for the patient and ought to be lowered.
- A patient with no or few mode switch events and no particular high rate atrial activity is probably doing fine.
- If a patient experiences a lot of mode switching and complains about abrupt rate transitions, increase the AMS base rate. (Note that not all pacemakers offer this particular feature.)

The reasons for using mode switching, especially with a programmable base rate are:

- it can prevent rapid ventricular response to high-rate intrinsic atrial activity (atrial tachyarrhythmias)
- it can make it easier for clinicians to manage patients with chronic or persistent atrial tachyarrhythmias, which could otherwise compromise effective dual-chamber pacing
- it allows patients with atrial tachyarrhythmias to derive the benefits of dual-chamber pacing most of the time, without experiencing the rapid ventricular response during atrial tachyarrhythmic episodes
- even patients who do not have documented atrial tachyarrhythmias may develop them, often without warning, so programming mode switching on can be a good safety net for patients. Mode switching only occurs when high atrial rates occur.

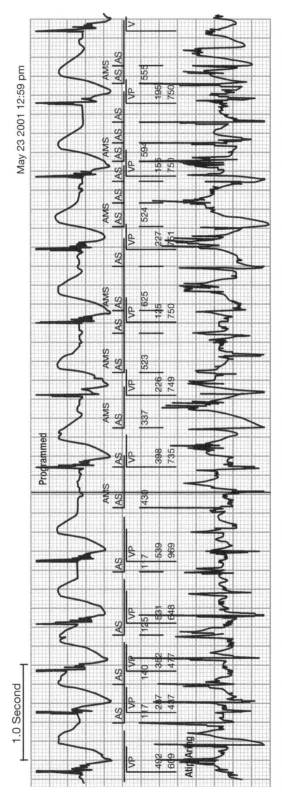

Fig. 13.1 The atrial electrogram (lower strip) documents the presence of atrial fibrillation. On the ECG, this rapid atrial rate caused some upper rate behavior until the AMS (auto mode switch) algorithm launched top-to-bottom vertical line) At that point, the pacemaker switched off the atrial channel and paced the ventricle while ignoring atrial activity. Atrial activity is still counted by the pacemakers, as attested by the annotations, since the algorithm makes its decisions based on counted atrial rates.

Hysteresis

The lower rate limit or base rate determines the rate at which the pacemaker will pace the heart in the absence of intrinsic activity. The hysteresis rate establishes the intrinsic rate that will cause the pacemaker to start pacing. In basic devices, a pacemaker programmed to a base rate of 70 ppm would pace at 70 ppm as soon as the intrinsic rate dropped to 69 bpm. By separating the base rate (pacing rate) from the hysteresis rate (sensing rate), it is possible to program the device so that it will indeed pace at 70 ppm (base rate) but *only when the patient's intrinsic rate falls below 60 bpm (hysteresis rate).*

Hysteresis became an important "new feature" decades ago when it was discovered that intrinsic activity is superior to paced activity and should therefore be encouraged. A programmed hysteresis rate allowed devices to stay inhibited, even at fairly low rates, to promote natural cardiac activity.

At the simplest level, programming hysteresis simply involves programming the rate the intrinsic heart rhythm must beat to avoid pacing. Setting a very low hysteresis rate encourages device inhibition and allows the intrinsic rate to emerge.

However, once the device starts pacing, it maintains the programmed base rate unless intrinsic activity at or above the programmed base rate inhibits pacing. In other words, the hysteresis rate only takes over when the device is inhibited (Fig. 13.2).

To further encourage intrinsic activity, a search function was added to hysteresis. For devices with "hysteresis with search," every so many cycles, the device extends one pacing cycle out to the hyster-esis rate. If intrinsic activity is sensed, then the device is inhibited and the hysteresis rate takes over. If no intrinsic event is sensed in the hysteresis search window, then the device resumes pacing at the programmed base rate. The search rate is essentially a way for the pacemaker to temporarily inhibit itself long enough to verify that no intrinsic activity close to the hysteresis rate is occurring.

For most pacemakers, clinicians may program a hysteresis rate and other parameters that govern the search function (how many cycles must elapse before a search cycle occurs).

While there is no specific "hysteresis histogram," clinicians can get a pretty good idea of how much hysteresis is affecting the pacemaker by looking at the amount (usually expressed as a percentage, sometimes as an absolute number) of time the device paced versus the amount it sensed. A large amount of sensed or intrinsic activity is desirable, if the patient has an adequate underlying rhythm. Obviously, some patients have very weak underlying rhythms and will be paced all or most of the time, no matter how hysteresis is programmed. But for patients with a somewhat adequate underlying rhythm – even if it is erratic – encouraging intrinsic activity is a good thing.

Hysteresis can also be programmed in an unusual way to help provide rate support for pacemaker patients who experience neurocardiogenic syncope. These patients have sudden fainting spells during which their blood pressure falls. An increased paced rate can contribute to the cardiac output in such a way as to help minimize the negative impact of a syncopal episode. In these patients, a relatively low

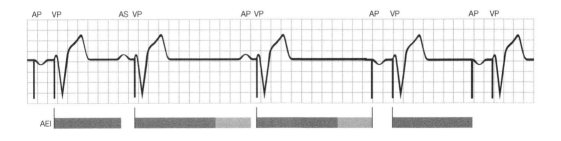

Hysteresis extension

Fig. 13.2 When hysteresis is programmed, the alert timing cycle is extended to look for intrinsic activity, which inhibits the pacemaker and resets the timing cycle. If no intrinsic activity is sensed during the hysteresis interval, the pacemaker resumes pacing at the programmed base rate. This can show up on a paced ECG as variations in the base rate.

hysteresis rate is selected, so that it only goes into effect when the patient experiences the rate drop-out typical of a syncopal spell. A slightly higher than normal base rate may be programmed so that when syncope occurs, pacing kicks in at a fairly rapid level to help boost cardiac output. For example, a pacemaker patient with known or suspected neurocardiogenic syncope might be programmed to a hysteresis rate of 40 bpm and a base rate of 90 ppm. Most of the time, the patient would not be paced because a hysteresis rate of 40 bpm is quite low. Even if the patient's own intrinsic rhythm remained in the 40s and 50s, he or she would not be paced. But if it ever did drop below 40, the programmed base rate would be activated and the patient would get sudden, relatively rapid rate support.

When evaluating hysteresis and how it's performing, there are some things to look for.

- Is the patient being paced most of the time? If there is reason to suspect that the patient's underlying intrinsic rhythm might be able to come through more often, the hysteresis rate can be lowered.
- If there is a good amount of sensed activity, that is a good thing providing the patient is getting the rate support needed. Make sure the patient is not symptomatic.
- Assess the patient's underlying rhythm and using clinical judgment, determine if the hysteresis rate can be lowered to allow more intrinsic rate control or if the underlying rhythm is too slow for the patient's needs.

The are various reasons for using hysteresis with search in pacemaker patients.

- For most pacemaker patients, hysteresis with search maximizes the time that the intrinsic rate will be in control. Since the intrinsic rate is always preferable to a paced rate (providing it is fast enough), optimizing intrinsic activity by helping to inhibit the device is important.
- For patients who have a good underlying rhythm that is erratic or not very slow, hysteresis allows them to experience the benefits of pacing without having to be paced most of the time.
- Hysteresis, in theory at least, can extend device longevity by helping to inhibit the device. (A device on standby uses far less energy than a device that is pacing. Likewise, a device that paces 50% of the time uses much less energy than one that paces

100% of the time.) Longer service life of a device means fewer surgeries and fewer replacements.
- For certain pacemaker patients with neurocardiogenic syncope and a good underlying rhythm, hysteresis programmed to a low rate with a somewhat higher base rate can help manage rate dropout events by jumping in with a relatively rapid paced response.

Ventricular intrinsic preference (VIP)

VIP technology was designed to minimize unnecessary right-ventricular pacing while still providing adequate ventricular pacing support. It is very similar to an earlier version of this feature known as autointrinsic conduction search (AICS). The VIP algorithm has a programmable search function. To search, the paced or sensed AV delay is automatically extended by a programmable duration at regular intervals (from every 30 seconds to every 30 minutes). If a sensed ventricular event (VS) occurs during the search interval or if three consecutive sensed ventricular events occur outside the search interval, the algorithm is activated, which means that the extended sensed and paced AV delay remains at the extended (longer) value. When no more intrinsic ventricular events occur in that extended AV delay for a programmable number of cycles, then the algorithm is deactivated and the sensed and paced AV delay are restored to originally programmed settings. The VIP algorithm works at rates up to 110 ppm (the older AICS algorithm worked at rates up to 90 ppm).

The purpose of these features is to minimize right-ventricular pacing when possible without interfering with the ventricular pacing support a patient might need. Since the algorithm is activated and deactivated very quickly, the patient experiences no obvious "rate bumps" during transitions.

PMT termination algorithms

Pacemaker-mediated tachycardia or PMT is a rapid heart rate which is not caused by the pacemaker, but which is facilitated by the presence of a pacemaker. For a patient to develop PMT, he or she needs a dual-chamber pacemaker, intact retrograde con-

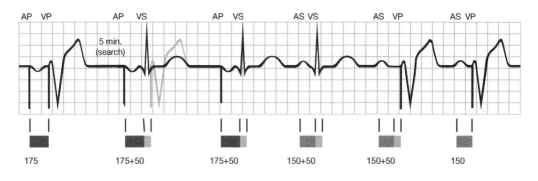

Fig. 13.3 The AICS algorithm extends the pacing cycle by a programmable delta (in this case 50 ms) to allow the device to sense any intrinsic activity. The faded paced ventricular event in the second complex is where the pacemaker would have paced without the intervening sensed event.

duction, and a precipitating cardiac event (usually a premature ventricular contraction or PVC). The most common causes of PMT are a PVC, the loss of atrial capture, or atrial undersensing. The pacemaker acts like a reentry path for the endless loop tachycardia.

Retrograde conduction refers to the heart's ability to conduct an electrical impulse backward (from ventricle to atrium or from apex upward) rather than forward. The normal conduction system of the healthy heart is a one-way street, with conduction moving forward only. Some patients, however, will have the ability to conduct an electrical impulse backward.

This requires a special substrate in the heart. Although there are no hard data on the subject, many pacemaker patients lack the ability to conduct in a retrograde direction and, as such, will not develop a PMT. The likelihood of retrograde conduction correlates with the general status of the patient's overall AV conduction system. Retrograde conduction is most common in pacemaker patients with intact AV conduction and sinus node dysfunction. Patients with complete heart block (no conduction through the AV node) have the lowest incidence of retrograde conduction, but just because an impulse cannot conduct forward through the AV node is no reason to assume it cannot conduct backward. In fact, some pacemaker patients with *complete heart block* will have retrograde conduction!

A PMT requires a trigger, i.e. an intrinsic cardiac event that creates an endless loop on the same order of a reentrant tachycardia. The most common PMT trigger is a PVC. PVCs are relatively common in both healthy and pacemaker patients. As mentioned before, other common triggers are any loss of AV synchrony, but particularly loss of atrial capture or atrial undersensing (i.e. inappropriate overpacing in the atrium).

The PVC or other event occurs, but instead of traveling forward along the conduction path, it goes backward. This causes a P wave (and resultant QRS) to become dissociated from the antegrade cardiac activity. This dissociated retrograde P wave falls in the atrial alert period, is sensed, and leads to a ventricular pacing output pulse. The circuit is complete and the cardiac activity now travels around the endless loop: forward from atrium to ventricle, then backward from ventricle to atrium. These signals get sensed by the atrial channel and cause a ventricular paced response (Fig. 13.5). Meanwhile, the patient's own heart may be beating intrinsically as well. The result is an endless-loop tachycardia sustained by the pacemaker.

A PMT requires a pacemaker with atrial sensing, and just about every approach to management of PMTs involves some way of temporarily turning off atrial sensing to break the endless loop. The atrial channel is not sensing true antegrade atrial activity, but rather retrograde signals.

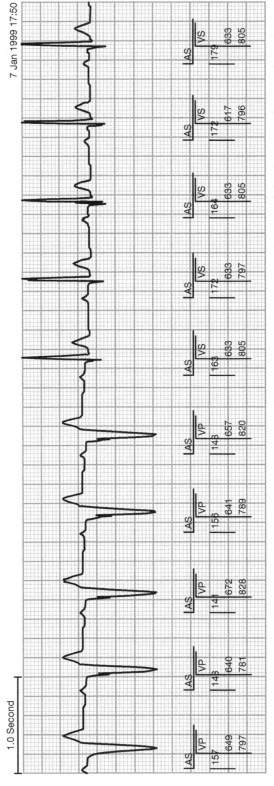

Fig. 13.4 This ECG shows AICS occurring in the middle of the strip with the first AS–VS complex annotated. The alert period was extended at this point and a ventricular event was sensed that normally would not have been able to prevail.

Even in patients who meet the conditions for potential PMTs, most PMTs can be avoided by programming a sufficiently long PVARP value (Fig. 13.6). The PVARP timing cycle defines how long the atrial channel will be unresponsive to atrial signals. Setting a PVARP value around 325 ms may prevent the majority of PMTs without compromising pacing therapy. Like any other pacemaker parameter setting, this is always a matter of clinical judgment.

Advanced pacemakers have other, special algorithms to manage PMTs. To program this sort of algorithm, it is first necessary to program a PMT detection rate, defined as the atrial rate at which the pacemaker will begin to evaluate whether or not a

PMT is in progress. A good standard value for the PMT detection rate is around 100 ppm. The first PMT algorithms used a simple rate criterion to assess the activity; if a lot of AS–VP state activity at or above the trigger rate occurred for a fixed number of cycles, the pacemaker counted that as a PMT and then withheld a ventricular output or extended the PVARP. If the rhythm was truly a PMT, these approaches would work to break it. (If, however, the high atrial rate was a native sinus rhythm, it would create a pause in the rhythm.)

The latest refinement in PMT algorithms came with AutoDetect. When the PMT detection rate trigger is reached, the system measures the VP–AS

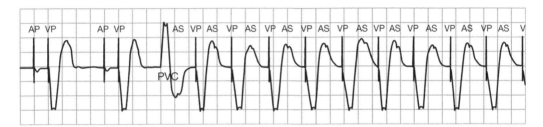

Fig. 13.5 A PVC occurs which launches a series of AS–VP events: intrinsic atrial activity (retrograde events, actually) prompting a ventricular response. A PMT can be very uncomfortable for the patient, who may complain of a racing or pounding heart.

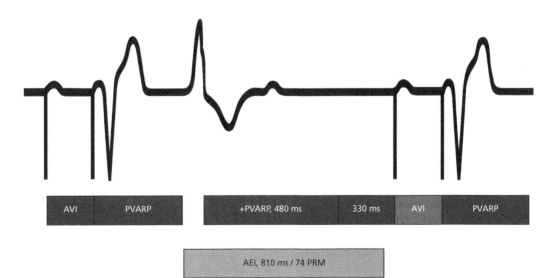

Fig. 13.6 One PMT option automatically extends the programmed PVARP value every time a PVC is detected. Since a PVC is a common trigger for a PMT, PVARP extension "blinds" the atrial channel during a time when a PMT is most likely to occur. When no PVC is detected, a more appropriate (shorter) PVARP prevails.

interval (not the AS–VP but the VP-to-AS) for eight cycles. If the VP–AS interval is stable over eight cycles, the rhythm is thought to be a likely PMT. On the ninth cycle, the system alters the AS–VP interval. In the case of a true PMT, an alteration in the AS–VP interval would not affect the stability of the VP–AS interval. If this occurs, the pacemaker diagnoses it as a "probable PMT."

On the other hand, if the pacemaker is just tracking a high sinus rhythm, a change in the AS–VP interval would indeed cause a change in the VP–AS interval. If that occurs, the pacemaker diagnoses "not PMT."

In the event that the system determines the rhythm to be a "probable PMT," it will withhold the ventricular output. Withholding a ventricular pacing output breaks the cycle of the PMT by removing the pacemaker's contribution to the vicious circle (Fig. 13.7).

The PMT algorithm also senses the next atrial event and 330 ms thereafter delivers an atrial output pulse. The 330 ms timing cycle gives the atrium enough time to recover from its physiological refractoriness, so that the atrial output is able to capture the atrium. Atrial capture makes the atrium refractory to incoming atrial signals, thus creating another break in the endless loop. This is sometimes called A-Pace on PMT.

While PMTs occurred more frequently in older pacing systems, they can still occur today. They were so common in earlier days that physicians routinely checked for retrograde conduction at implant in order to program the device initially. Today, PMT algorithms and an adequately programmed PVARP setting can prevent many PMTs.

Nevertheless, it is good clinical practice to check for retrograde conduction during follow-up sessions, particularly if there is evidence of a disproportionately high percentage of AS–VP complexes at relatively high rates. For patients who complain about palpitations or for whom diagnostic counters make the clinician suspect PMTs, retrograde conduction should be tested. Bear in mind that retrograde conduction can come and go; patients who do not have evidence of retrograde conduction at one follow-up session may develop it later on.

To assess retrograde conduction in a dual-chamber pacemaker patient, temporarily program the rate higher than the patient's intrinsic atrial rate.

This forces pacing. Then temporarily program the pacemaker to the VVI mode and check the surface ECG for any deformation of the S–T segment of the strip. A deformity in the S–T segment indicates retrograde conduction. If the pacemaker allows simultaneous atrial telemetry while in this state (VVI mode), check the atrial channel to see if any atrial activity is occurring (retrograde P waves). Although this method is not exact and certainly not foolproof, it can determine retrograde conduction in many pacemaker patients. For other patients, the best strategy is to assume that the patient has the potential to develop PMTs, even if retrograde conduction cannot be established conclusively.

The following are reasons for using a PMT termination algorithm.

- Many (but not all) dual-chamber pacemaker patients have the conditions needed to experience a PMT. If a PMT is suspected or even possible, these algorithms can help pre-empt them.
- People with no evidence of retrograde conduction may still have it or may develop it without warning.
- Suspect PMTs in any patients with lots of AS–VP activity at fairly high rates. A PMT termination algorithm can help prevent this.
- For patients who complain about palpitations, or a racing heart, it is possible they are having PMTs rather than another form of tachycardia. The PMT algorithm can provide relief.

Auto Rest Rate

The "perfect pacemaker" is the one that most accurately and consistently mimics the activities of the healthy heart. Healthy hearts normally increase their rate during exertion (which the pacemaker mimics with rate response) and decrease their rate during periods of rest and sleep. For many years, pacemakers offered a programmable base rate that could increase with activity, but which did not decrease when the patient went to sleep. Some patients found their "day rates" were far too rapid to be comfortable during sleep.

The earliest approach to this problem of rate slow-down at night (or rest) was to allow the pacemaker to have time-dependent rates, so that the pacing rate automatically decreased at a certain clock time. While this worked for patients who kept to

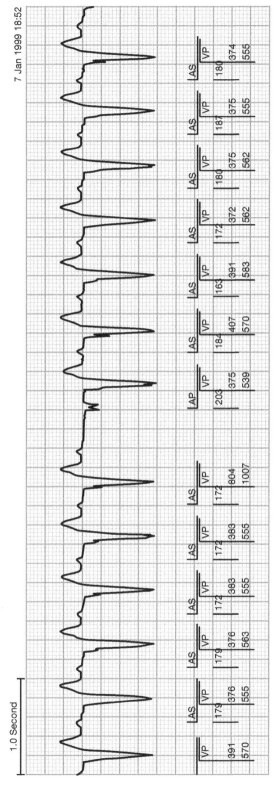

Fig. 13.7 This pacemaker has diagnosed the activity as a "probable PMT" and in about the middle of the strip has withheld a ventricular output. This breaks the cycle (as evidenced by the AP–VP event) and restores AS–VP pacing at a slower rate.

strict bedtimes, for patients with erratic schedules or those who traveled to other time zones, it sometimes resulted in rates that slowed when the patient was awake or that kept pacing at the more rapid rate as the patient was trying to go to sleep.

Auto Rest Rate was instituted to allow the patient's activity level to determine when the rate slowdown would occur. Auto Rest Rate is only available in pacemakers with an activity sensor, although the sensor may be programmed to PASSIVE rather than active (if desired). This function is programmable by setting a special rest rate value, which is a rate lower than the base rate. The rest rate should be the rate the pacemaker should pace the heart while the patient is asleep.

In theory, the Auto Rest Rate imposes a programmable rest rate (which should be programmed to a value lower than the programmed base rate) whenever the pacemaker (based on activity levels) has determined that the patient is asleep. It looks at inactivity measured over a period of 15 or 20 min rather than brief spells of inactivity.

While the Auto Rest Rate does rely on activity to start and stop the rest rate, it does not take direct sensor data. Instead, it has an algorithm that allows the pacemaker to compare short-term sensor activity data to long-term data compiled over the past 7 days. In that way, the pacemaker will not be fooled by brief spells of inactivity, nor will it regard long-term bedridden behavior as true sleep.

There are various reasons for programming the Auto Rest Rate.

- Most patients find it more comfortable to sleep when the pacemaker is not pacing their hearts at 60 or 70 ppm. This type of pacing may actually keep them awake.
- The Auto Rest Rate does not depend on clock times and allows the patient freedom to change his or her sleep schedule.
- The Auto Rest Rate is based on activity rather than clock time, so it never needs to be reset with daylight savings time, travel, or special schedules.
- By mimicking the healthy heart, it gives patients a more natural sleep/wake cycle and may help certain pacemaker patients get more or better-quality sleep.

Conclusion

Special features offer the clinician some very powerful tools to improve diagnostic ability, streamline follow-up, and provide better therapy. But the key to deriving maximum benefit from special features is to match the right patient with the right features. To do that, the theoretical purpose of the special feature as well as the practical knowledge to activate it and use it need to be understood. Experienced pacemaker practitioners get very adept at these settings and can fine-tune parameters to meet a wide variety of patient needs, but even the clinician who only occasionally sees a pacemaker patient should be aware of some of the advanced features available.

Some of these features may create unusual patterns on the rhythm strips that defy explanation unless it is realized that a special algorithm is in effect. Furthermore, knowing about the availability of some of these features in the latest pacemakers may help to address the special needs or complaints of pacemaker patients.

While these sophisticated features may seem complicated, they are designed to be intuitively understood and easy to program. In fact, many are semi-automatic if not totally automatic (you may have to program something on or adjust one or two settings). And, in truth, even pacemaker experts rarely program all of the available parameters on a device except in the most unusual cases.

Further reading

Ammirati F, Colivicchi F, Toscano S *et al.* DDD pacing with rate drop response function versus DDDI with rate hysteresis pacing for cardioinhibitory vasovagal syncope. *PACE* 1998; **21** (11 Part 2): 2178–81.

Levine PA. *Guidelines to the Routine Evaluation, Programming and Follow-up of the Patient with an Implanted Dual-Chamber Rate-Modulated Pacing System.* Sylmar, CA: St Jude Medical, 2003.

Morris-Thurgood J, Chiang CM, Rochelle J *et al.* A rate-responsive pacemaker that physiologically reduces pacing rates at rest. *PACE* 1994; **17** (11 Part 2): 1928–32.

Provenier F, Jordaens L, Verstraeten T *et al.* The automatic mode switch function in successive generations of minute-ventilation sensing dual-chamber rate-responsive pacemakers. *PACE* 1994; **17** (11 Part 2): 1913–19.

Schuchert A, van Langen H, Michels K *et al.* DDD(R) pacing with automatic mode switch in patients with paroxysmal atrial fibrillation following AV nodal ablation. *Cardiology* 1997; **88**: 323–7.

Sutton R. How and when to pace in vasovagal syncope. *J Cardiovasc Electrophysiol* 2002; **13** (1 Suppl): S14–S16.

Yue AM, Thomas RD. Neurocardiogenic syncope due to recurrent tonsillar carcinoma: successful treatment by dual-chamber cardiac pacing with rate hysteresis. *PACE* 2002; **25**: 121–2.

The nuts and bolts of special features

- The latest pacemakers have the latest features; in clinical practice, you will be dealing with old and new pacemakers, so not all devices will have all of the latest features.
- While many companies offer devices with similar special features, they often use different terminology and may work slightly differently. It is always a good idea to check the device manual or take advantage of training materials from the various manufacturers.
- Auto Mode Switching or AMS turns off the atrial channel in the presence of high rate atrial activity, so that there is no rapid ventricular response. The AMS base rate allows an interim rate (higher than the base rate) during AMS episodes, to prevent abrupt rate decreases that patients often report as uncomfortable and even distressing.
- Hysteresis encourages intrinsic conduction by allowing the native activity to dominate when it occurs at a certain level (lower than the base rate but above a programmable hysteresis rate). The search function allows the device to periodically look for intrinsic events at the hysteresis rate so that intrinsic conduction will prevail.
- Ventricular intrinsic preference and its predecessor autointrinsic conduction search periodically lengthen the sensed or paced AV delay to extend the ventricular alert period; this is another way the device can search out intrinsic (in this case, ventricular) activity.
- The goal of ventricular intrinsic preference is to minimize unnecessary right-ventricular pacing without denying the patient the benefit of adequate ventricular rate support.
- PMT termination algorithms help break the endless cycle of PMT in pacemaker patients by pacing in a certain way when a PMT is detected.
- To have a PMT a patient needs three things: a dual-chamber pacemaker, intact retrograde conduction, and a triggering event, usually a premature ventricular contraction (PVC). PMT works like an endless-loop tachycardia, but it is facilitated (not caused) by the pacemaker.
- If the PMT algorithm determines that a rapid ventricular rate is actually a PMT, then it inhibits a precisely timed ventricular output pulse and delivers an atrial output pulse 330 ms after the last atrial sensed event. These two things are each sufficient on their own to break the endless loop.
- Another way to avoid PMTs in most patients is to program a long PVARP. For most patients, a PVARP of 325 ms is sufficient to prevent most PMTs.
- Auto Rest Rate mimics the normal rate decrease of the healthy heart during sleep by using the activity sensor to determine when a patient is asleep and reducing the rate at such times to the programmed rest rate. The best rest rates are those that depend on an activity sensor algorithm rather than clock time since many patients do not adhere to a strict sleep/wake schedule.

CHAPTER 14

Systematic follow-up

There are many goals to pacemaker follow-up. Among other things, pacemaker follow-up should verify proper operation of the pacemaker, maximize device longevity, optimize the programmed parameter settings, detect the end of service, troubleshoot any known or unknown problems, and establish a record of information about the session. Another goal of pacemaker follow-up is to minimize patient anxiety! In order to meet these multiple objectives and to alleviate clinician anxiety in the process, pacemaker follow-up needs to be systematic.

Systematic pacemaker follow-up means an established routine of steps that are carried out during follow-up. Systematic follow-up both streamlines follow-up and increases the likelihood that obscure problems are detected, even in cases where the patient has no symptoms.

Pacemaker patients require regular and consistent follow-up for a variety of reasons.

- First and foremost, a pacemaker is a mechanical device with a finite (battery-controlled) lifespan. Pacemaker follow-up verifies that the device is operating and ascertains the best time for *device replacement* as the battery exhausts itself.
- Second, follow-up gives the clinician a chance to *fine-tune the pacing prescription* to meet the patient's changing physical condition, new diagnoses, added or discontinued drugs, and other factors that may influence the optimal setting of the various programmable parameters.
- Third, pacemaker follow-up is a chance for the clinicians to download information stored in the pacemaker to *keep a record* of the patient's condition.
- Last and most infrequently, pacemaker follow-up can help the clinician detect and *troubleshoot problems*, sometimes before the patient becomes symptomatic.

Beyond these obvious clinical reasons, pacemaker follow-up helps clinics stay in touch with pacemaker patients. While pacemaker recalls are rare (especially considering the millions of pacemaker patients who have devices that can be expected to function for years without any trouble at all), they can happen. In such cases, it is imperative for the doctor or clinic to be able to notify patients who might have the affected device. Patients who routinely report for follow-up visits not only have the best chance to get optimal pacing therapy, they are most likely to get timely information in the unlikely event there is some concern over their device.

The official ACC/AHA/HRS *Guidelines on Pacemakers* states that pacemaker follow-up is influenced by a variety of factors, including age and condition of the patient, whether or not the doctor is also treating the patient for other conditions, the type of pacing system in place, and geographical location. In this last regard, it is increasingly recognized that visits to the follow-up clinic represent a considerable hardship to some patients, particularly those who live in remote locations or for whom there is no nearby doctor. All of these factors must be assessed when a follow-up schedule is determined.

In the United States, the Health Care Financing Administration (HCFA) set forth its guidelines in 1984. While individual factors may impact or override this, HCFA recommends that single-chamber pacemakers be followed twice in the first 6 months post-implant and then every 12 months thereafter. Dual-chamber pacemakers should likewise be checked twice in the first 6 months post-implant and then every 6 months thereafter.

In addition, the guidelines allow at least some of these follow-up sessions to be in the form of transtelephonic monitoring (TTM). TTM was one of the earliest forms of what is today known as "remote patient monitoring." In this very popular forerunner of "telemedicine," patients can download pacemaker information over an ordinary phone line for evaluation by a service center. TTM can merely accept information from the pacemaker; it cannot reprogram the device. Nevertheless, for patients in otherwise good health or for whom a trip to the clinic for a check-up represents a major inconvenience, TTM can serve as an excellent method to keep an eye on the pacemaker without necessitating a full follow-up.

One challenge to the goal of systematic follow-up is that the average pacemaker clinic sees many different models of pacemakers. These different devices may require different programmers and the physical challenge of setting up multiple programmers over the course of a pacemaker clinic. Older devices lack some of the sophisticated features of today's systems, which may mandate different programming tactics. (For example, some pacemakers encountered in clinical practice will not offer mode switching, which can make it difficult to manage a patient with persistent atrial tachyarrhythmias.) Manufacturers may use slightly different terminology in similar features, so that a good follow-up clinician has to learn to "speak Medtronic" as fluently as he can "speak St Jude Medical." In some ways, learning multiple devices is similar to mastering several different software programs on the computer.

If you are following a patient with a relatively new pacemaker, you probably can take advantage of a one-button follow-up feature which runs through a systematic follow-up sequence. These features are a great convenience and assure that no step is ever inadvertently overlooked or omitted. On the other hand, most pacemaker clinics see an abundance of patients with much older devices that require the clinicians to walk through the steps one-by-one.

For that reason and for didactic purposes, this book is going to proceed through the various steps in a systematic follow-up. Realize that in newer devices, there may be automated choices that will carry out the steps for you.

Step one: the patient interview

The key component in any pacing system is not the pulse generator or the lead, but the patient. Begin by asking how the patient is feeling, paying special attention to any symptoms that might relate to decreased cardiac output. Since most pacemaker patients are geriatric (85% of all pacemaker patients are 64 years old or older), they are likely to have other illnesses. This means that not every symptom they report will relate to the pacemaker. (Be aware that it is not uncommon, especially for new pacemaker patients, to attribute every new ache and pain to the pacemaker.)

In the patient interview, look for complaints that could mean the patient is experiencing impaired cardiac output. Symptoms that could relate to decreased cardiac output include:
• dizziness
• palpitations, a "racing heart," pounding in the chest
• shortness of breath
• feeling faint, woozy, light-headed
• fatigue.

Associated signs include changes in skin color, respiratory rate, and edema. Such information should be carefully noted in the file. Signs and symptoms of decreased cardiac output are reasons to suspect that the pacemaker is not performing as well as it ought or that the settings are not right for that particular patient.

Next, examine the implant site for signs of redness, infection, or erosion. The patient's neck veins should be evaluated for distention. The patient's heart rate, blood pressure, and heart and lung sounds should be checked.

Before you check the patient with the programmer, it is important to assess the level of what is called "pacemaker dependency" (Table 14.1). If a patient is significantly pacemaker dependent, only a physician who is familiar with pacemaker programming should handle the follow-up. For patients who are not severely pacemaker dependent, it is routine practice to allow an associated professional or a physician to handle follow-up. This becomes a matter of clinical judgment.

Table 14.1 Pacemaker dependency

Escape rhythm	Degree of dependency
No escape rhythm	Total
Ventricular tachyarrhythmias	Total
Complete AV block (with AF or sinus rhythm)	Substantial
Sinus bradycardia < 30 bpm	Moderate
Lesser degree of AV block	Moderate
Regular sinus rhythm at a rate ≥ 50 bpm	Not dependent

The reason for concern over pacemaker dependency is that pacemaker follow-up routinely involves threshold and sensing testing, both of which may require the clinician to try to force the patient's intrinsic rhythm to break through and to temporarily suspend normal pacemaker operation. Those who do not depend on the pacemaker tolerate these tests well, but pacemaker-dependent people may experience symptoms during such tests. In the event that a patient is dependent on the pacemaker to some degree, good clinical judgment is required to weigh the benefits of routine follow-up testing against the risks of temporarily suspending normal pacemaker operation. That is not a decision for a pacemaker novice to make!

Some pacing clinics sticker or otherwise color-code the files of patients who have been found to be pacemaker dependent. While pacemaker dependency may not be a static state, most clinicians agree that any patient once determined to be pacemaker dependent should always be treated as dependent thereafter.

There may not always be sufficient information available to assess the degree of pacemaker dependency. In such cases, it is wise to be on the lookout for a very slow escape rhythm or signs of heart block and ventricular tachyarrhythmias, all of which signal that certain types of testing in which the pacemaker might be temporarily programmed off or to very subnormal settings should be avoided.

Step two: using the programmer, get a running ECG and interrogate the device to get the programmed settings

Pacemaker follow-up requires a programmer or so-called patient care system, the table-top proprietary computer that allows you to communicate with the implanted device. Most pacemaker clinics have many different programmers available. It is important to know the right programmer to use. Unfortunately, there is no universal compatibility when it comes to pacemaker programmers. Not only do manufacturers' programmers only work on devices from that manufacturer, some manufacturers may have more than one programmer to accommodate several different devices. In recent years, most pacemaker manufacturers have made tremendous strides in consolidating the programming function so that the latest generation of programmers is "backward-compatible" with most older devices. Nevertheless, it is still not unusual in clinical practice to run into the need to use a less-familiar programmer from time to time.

If the patient is a regular at the clinic, the patient file should contain enough information on the pacemaker to find the proper programmer. For pacemakers of relatively recent vintage from one of the "big three" major manufacturers, it is safe to use the main programmer from that manufacturer. (For example, a patient with a St Jude Medical Victory® pacemaker can be programmed with the latest patient care system from St Jude Medical, the Merlin®.)

There are other ways to ascertain the type of pacemaker.

- Ask the patient for the pacemaker ID card that he should have received from the manufacturer. Be sure to check the year; if the patient has had several replacement generators, he may not be carrying the latest ID card.
- If the patient does not have an ID card, his regular physician, referring cardiologist, or even family members may know the device manufacturer.
- In the event that the information cannot be obtained in this way, a chest X-ray will reveal the size and shape of the pacemaker along with an X-ray ID tag. People very familiar with pacemakers can often identify a device quickly in this way. Most manufacturers make ID charts or posters showing X-ray images of their devices, which can then be matched against the radiograph of the patient.
- If you can read the ID tag, most pacemaker representatives and all technical hotlines have a complete reference to identify devices by the ID. In addition, manufacturers are required to keep records of patients who receive their devices.
- It's only really important to know the manufacturer to match the programmer to the pacemaker. Once you have the right company's programmer in place, most modern devices will self-identify.

There is a risk involved in using the wrong programmer (from a different company) for an implanted pacemaker. It will not work, but it may actually interfere with the implanted pacemaker. For that reason, it is important to take all necessary steps to assure that the proper programmer is used.

Once you have the right programmer in place, begin by attaching the stick-on electrodes to the patient for the ECG portion of the follow-up. Some newer devices offer wireless ECGs and wireless telemetry, so there is no need to attach electrodes. Using the programmer's ECG capability (common to all programmers), obtain a free-running ECG. This ECG should be evaluated using the basic ECG evaluation approach.

- Is there capture?
- Is there sensing?
- What is the patient's underlying rhythm?

The ECG should be saved as part of documentation of the visit. Medicare and other guidelines mandate these records, which should be recorded in the patient's chart. One key element of successful pacemaker follow-up is meticulous attention to documentation!

Once the ECG is obtained, the device can be addressed. If you have a relatively new pacemaker, you may be able to use an automatic follow-up sequence, which allows for one-button or otherwise streamlined operation. This single button should be accessible directly on the programmer. Older devices may not permit this step and will require the individual activation of a sequence.

After an initial 30-second ECG is obtained, a magnet should be placed over the implanted pulse generator. A magnet will close the magnet switch in the device and induce magnet mode. Magnet mode varies by manufacturer, and even by device, but generally involves asynchronous pacing (AOO, VOO or DOO mode). Asynchronous pacing will override the patient's intrinsic rhythm and put pacemaker spikes on the ECG, making it easier for the clinician to verify proper function of the device. Magnet mode can also provide information to help assess battery state and replacement indicators. After a 30-second magnet strip is obtained for the chart, run another 30-second non-magnet ECG strip.

During programming, the clinician must establish telemetry with the implanted device. For older devices, the programmer wand (the portion of the programmer that looks most like a TV remote control) is placed over the implanted device. For the newer generation of wireless devices, this step may not be necessary as the programmer can communicate wirelessly with the implanted system.

Whether accessed through an automated sequence or as an individual step, the first step in the process is interrogation (sometimes called inquiry). With communication established (wirelessly or via the programmer wand), press the button on the programmer for automated follow-up or for interrogation. The programmer makes contact with the device and in a few moments, the programmer screen will reveal device identification information (model number), the currently programmed settings for the parameters, and sometimes other information.

It is crucial that this information be printed out. Most programmers today have a built-in printer that can be easily accessed from a button on the programmer. Print out the programmed parameters as they were at the start of the follow-up session. It is important for the follow-up that you know exactly how the device was programmed and how it is supposed to be operating for you to verify its proper operation!

Obtain telemetry to get information on pacing system parameters, in particular lead impedance. Again, in more automated systems, this may be part of the interrogation step. The most crucial value in this series for routine follow-up is the lead impedance value.

Lead impedance values are not programmable, and they can be expected to fluctuate somewhat over time. Many pacemakers have the ability to store past lead impedance values in memory so that a current value can be quickly compared to previous values, in numeric or graphic format. In the event of an older pacemaker, lead impedance values should be recorded in the patient's chart at each and every follow-up session.

Lead impedance values can vary considerably from patient to patient and even over time in a single patient. The key to evaluating this parameter is not looking for a specific value, but rather looking for significant changes. As a rule of thumb, a sharp increase in lead impedance ($> 200 \, \Omega$) may be indicative of a lead fracture, i.e. a break in the lead that compromises its ability to pace and sense properly. Likewise, a dramatic decrease in lead impedance (again, $> 200 \, \Omega$) may indicate an insulation break.

Thus, it is almost always impossible to look at one lead impedance value in isolation and assign it any sort of diagnostic value. After all, if lead impedance is 700 Ω, that does not tell you much. On the other hand, if lead impedance is 700 Ω now, but at last follow-up, lead impedance was just 300 Ω, that indicates a problem. In fact, it suggests that the lead's conductor coil is broken.

If you get a dramatic change (> 200 Ω) in lead impedance value, follow these steps.

- Repeat the telemetry to get a second reading to confirm.
- Lead problems are best viewed on a radiograph. A chest X-ray is the logical next step to visualize what might be wrong with the lead.
- Check the paced ECG to see if there is unusual activity. Lead problems can sometimes result in sensing or pacing abnormalities.
- A normal-looking radiograph and a normal paced ECG in the presence of sharp impedance changes mandates close surveillance of the patient. A lead problem may be in the works.
- A pacing specialist should be consulted if there is a broken or severely compromised lead. In most cases, a new lead will have to be implanted.

Step three: download diagnostics

Most pacemakers offer a wealth of counters and other functions that constantly record cardiac activity. These counters then report their data in bar charts, tables, graphs, or numerical lists. In fact, many pacemaker programmers will offer redundant diagnostic counters in a choice of formats, i.e. you can see the same information in numerical or chart form. Begin with a printout of the FastPath™ Summary or top-level overview of programmed parameter settings. Then retrieve the diagnostic information.

Diagnostic data vary by pacemaker, but should always be accessed and evaluated during follow-up. The great value of diagnostic data is that they show the clinician exactly (and, in contrast to the patient's own reports, objectively) how the pacemaker and the patient have been interacting since the last follow-up.

While terminology may differ by manufacturer and model, here are the main types of diagnostic data that are available.

- **Heart rate histogram.** This is useful to see what rates the patient has been experiencing since the last follow-up. These rates should be appropriate for the patient's lifestyle. The rate distribution should be appropriate.
- **Event histogram.** This is a quick reference type of histogram which states pacing states by percentages without regard to rates. The pacing states should be appropriate for the patient's condition. (For example, a patient with sick sinus syndrome should not have a lot of AS–VP activity.) A lot of PVCs can be a red flag (although a small number of PVCs are no cause for alarm).
- **AT/AF histograms** show how frequently high intrinsic atrial rates were detected and how the pacemaker responded. This screen will show AT/AF burden in percentage, peak A rate histograms, and an AT/AF log with the date, time, maximum rate, and duration of the latest AT/AF episodes. If the patient has no atrial tachyarrhythmias, there may be nothing to see on this diagnostic report. On the other hand, for patients with high atrial rates, this diagnostic information can reveal how often atrial tachyarrhythmias are occurring, their rates (whether they are moderate or dangerously fast) and can help troubleshoot problems that can occur when AT overlaps with sinus tachycardia.
- **AF Suppression™ diagnostics** report how this particular algorithm performed, how often it went into effect, and under what conditions.
- **Stored EGMs.** Many modern pacemakers have the capacity to store intracardiac EGMs in memory for subsequent download; the memory capacity in some pacemakers allows for many minutes of such recordings. Clinicians can program "triggers" or gating events that initiate the memory to start recording an EGM, which is stored in memory. EGMs should be downloaded and evaluated during follow-up. Some commonly programmed stored EGM triggers are high-rate atrial activity, mode switch events, and PVCs. While stored EGMs are easily the most valuable diagnostic tool in the toolkit, the limited memory capacity of the implantable device means that sometimes the device has to overwrite old EGMs to store new EGMs. As a result, not all of the EGMs that trigger a recording will be available for download. Most devices store EGMs on the "first in, first out" sys-

tem, meaning the newest information overwrites the oldest once the memory is maxed out. Very recent devices from St Jude Medical offer preferential EGM storage, which allows the clinician to set up guidelines for overwriting EGMs once the memory is full.

• **Patient-triggered stored EGMs.** In addition to stored EGMs that are automatically recorded when a triggering event occurs, some devices allow the patient to initiate a recording. This feature is only useful when the patient is willing and able to comply with the system, which requires him to record an EGM whenever he experiences a "dizzy spell" or other event. For patients bothered by certain symptoms, patient-triggered stored EGMs can be very useful in getting a problem to "go on the record."

Downloading these diagnostics now (and printing them out) provides a complete, documented record of how the device and patient behaved since the last follow-up. It is crucial to print out this information, since it is not necessarily otherwise stored.

Many diagnostic counters are set up to overwrite the oldest records when they get full. In this way, the clinician only has access to the latest information. Printed diagnostics from a follow-up session can be useful historical records for long-term trends or comparison.

When looking over the diagnostic data, the clinician should run through the following systematic questions.

1 *Are the diagnostic data consistent with the programmed settings?* For instance, if mode switching is programmed on, there should not be periods of high-rate atrial activity followed by rapid ventricular response. If AF Suppression™ is on, there should be atrial pacing.

2 *Is there anything unusual in the diagnostics?* Unusual data include an unusually large amount of a certain type of activity (for instance, a particularly high PVC count), large counts of certain algorithms (for instance, large number of mode switch episodes) or a lot of high-rate activity. Note that some unusual patterns in the diagnostics may not be indicative of anything wrong (for instance, almost exclusively AS–VP pacing).

3 *Are all programmed algorithms functioning appropriately?* Consider how the device is set and evaluate

such things as rate response, hysteresis, and PMT termination algorithms.

4 *Are there clues in the diagnostics of possible problems or things that might require troubleshooting?* Such things include:
   (a) lots of high-rate atrial activity with rapid ventricular response (this may be addressed by mode switching or the AF Suppression™ algorithm)
   (b) lots of high-rate atrial activity, regardless of ventricular response (mode switching or the AF Suppression™ algorithm should be considered)
   (c) sensor-driven rates that seem excessively high for the patient's lifestyle (sensor settings may be too aggressive)
   (d) anything that differs significantly from previous diagnostic counters (which may indicate that a problem has been solved or that a new one is emerging)
   (e) anything markedly unusual.

As a general recommendation, clear the counters (zero them out) after you print out the information. This allows the diagnostic functions to track events that happened at the follow-up session (which is sometimes useful) and also assures that counters are cleared before the patient leaves. It is important to clear the diagnostic counters after each and every follow-up session to provide the most accurate diagnostic data for the next clinician. If counters are not cleared, the next several months worth of activity will be diluted in the old data and have less interpretative value.

Some clinicians may prefer to go through the various diagnostic counters as they progress through systematic follow-up. It is more important that a clinician develop a solid, methodical system than the actual sequence of the steps. It is recommended, however, that diagnostics be downloaded early in the process as well as consulted later.

Keep the printouts of the diagnostic data handy in the patient's chart as the follow-up progresses. As the various steps unfold, it may become important to consult with the diagnostic counters to better understand certain types of pacemaker behavior.

Step four: capture threshold testing

If you are following a pacemaker with the AutoCapture™ pacing systems, you do not need to perform a separate capture threshold test. You may download the Capture Threshold Monitoring diagnostics to see how capture has been maintained and note threshold variations. Because AutoCapture™ pacing systems are automatic, self-regulating systems, you do not need to assess a capture threshold value and then determine a safety margin for proper programming.

Other pacemakers offer automatic or semi-automatic capture threshold testing which allows you to activate a test sequence with just one or two simple steps.

The theory behind capture threshold testing is the step-down sequence. A pacing output is selected at which there is known capture. The pacing output value is then decreased in small increments and retested until capture is lost. At the point capture is lost, the sequence is stepped up until capture is achieved. The value at which capture is restored after being lost becomes the "capture threshold" (Fig. 14.1). In older pacemaker systems, this test has to be done manually (or at least with a few semi-automatic steps). When doing step-down testing, continuous ECG monitoring is essential.

For testing capture in a single-chamber pacing system, program the base rate to a rate slightly higher than the patient's intrinsic rhythm and observe the ECG. If there is capture (spikes followed by depolarizations), the system is probably operating correctly.

In dual-chamber systems, it is important to first determine what sort of pacing events are occurring. Look at the initial running ECG that was obtained at the outset or check diagnostic counters to see the dominant pacing states. (It is rare to get only one type of pacing, but there is usually one state that occurs more frequently than the others.)

AP–VP: If the pacemaker is mostly pacing in both atrium and ventricle, the step-down capture tests are done just as they would be done in a single-chamber system. Assess one chamber, then the other. There is no particular recommended order.

AS–VS: In this dual-chamber pacing state, the pacemaker is mostly inhibited with occasional paced events. Start by programming the rate higher than the patient's own rate and program a long AV delay value. This should result in AP–VP or AP–VS pacing, that is the atrium is paced and the ventricle responds, whether on its own or by a paced beat. Now test the atrium for the capture threshold, using the step-down technique described for single-chamber systems. When atrial capture is lost, it will not only be evident on the ECG, there will also be no more ventricular sensed events (when atrial capture is lost, there is nothing to conduct to the ventricles). The only ventricular activity after the loss of atrial capture is a ventricular paced event which, in fact, confirms the true loss of atrial capture. Note the atrial threshold value.

Move to the ventricle by leaving a rate that is high enough to override the intrinsic rhythm, but this time program a short AV delay. It is not unusual to opt for the shortest available AV delay setting for this temporary test. (The goal is to avoid conduction.) Gradually step-down the ventricular pulse amplitude until ventricular capture is lost. Again, be sure to document the settings. Double the pulse amplitude of the capture threshold to program the conventional safety margin.

AS–VP: In this pacing state, there is sinus rhythm but it does not conduct reliably to the ventricle, so the ventricular response is generally a paced beat. Start with the atrial capture threshold test by programming to a base rate that overdrives the patient's intrinsic rhythm. Do not, however, exceed 100 ppm for atrial threshold testing. It may not be possible to pace faster than the patient's own atrial rhythm and stay under 100 ppm. If that is the case and the pacemaker was in DDI mode, temporarily program the mode to DDD. This should result in stable AP–VP pacing. If it does not, an experienced pacing clinician should evaluate the patient and determine if and how to conduct the atrial threshold test.

Assuming the DDD reprogramming results in stable AP–VP pacing, test the atrium using the step-down technique until capture is lost. The resulting rhythm should include runs of AS–VP pacing. Do not be overly concerned if the rhythm is erratic. Note the atrial threshold and program twice the pulse amplitude to achieve the conventional safety margin.

The ventricular threshold can be tested in the straightforward manner. Start with paced ventricular activity, step-down the amplitude until capture is lost, and then document the value. To program the final settings, program a value at least twice the pulse amplitude of the documented capture threshold.

If the currently programmed settings are appropriate, there is no need to do anything. However,

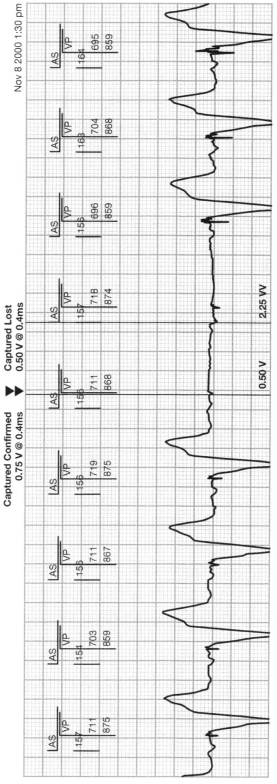

Fig. 14.1 Ventricular threshold test in a patient with a dual-chamber pacemaker system and AV nodal block. Capture is lost in the ventricle at the first line (note the VP annotation, indicating an output was delivered with no corresponding ventricular response) and restored two complexes later. The device notes the values at which capture was lost and restored.

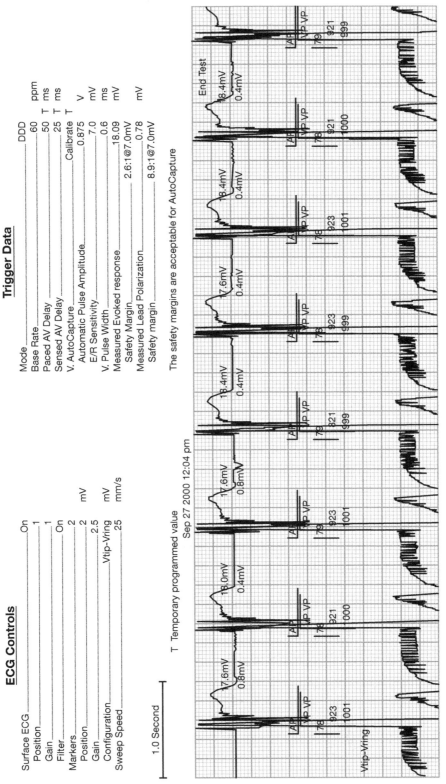

ECG Controls

Surface ECG	On
Position	1
Gain	1
Filter	On
Markers	2 mV
Position	2
Gain	2.5
Configuration	Vtip-Vring mV
Sweep Speed	25 mm/s

T Temporary programmed value

Sep 27 2000 12:04 pm

1.0 Second

Trigger Data

Mode	DDD	
Base Rate	60	ppm
Paced AV Delay	50	T ms
Sensed AV Delay	25	T ms
V. AutoCapture	Calibrate	T
Automatic Pulse Amplitude	0.875	V
E/R Sensitivity	7.0	mV
V. Pulse Width	0.6	ms
Measured Evoked response	18.09	mV
Safety Margin	2.6:1@7.0mV	
Measured Lead Polarization	0.78	
Safety margin	8.9:1@7.0mV	mV

The safety margins are acceptable for AutoCapture

Fig. 14.2 Ventricular evoked response sensitivity test from an AutoCapture™ pacing system.

it may be necessary to adjust the output settings to achieve capture or to assure an adequate safety margin. (In AutoCapture™ pacing systems, this is not necessary.)

Some pacemakers will offer to draw a strength–duration curve to show all of the options for the best output settings. The strength–duration curve is essentially a chart of all the combinations of pulse amplitude/pulse width values that would work to capture the heart. It shows that at very short pulse widths, very high pulse amplitudes are needed to capture the heart. As the pulse width extends, less and less pulse amplitude is needed to get capture. At a certain point, the graph flattens out, showing that there is a specific minimum voltage that is required for capture, regardless of how long the pulse width might be prolonged. While the strength–duration curve is a useful function, there is no need to print it out or add it to the patient's chart. It's primarily a reference tool.

Step five: sensing threshold testing

The next step is to assess the sensing function of the pacemaker by conducting a sensing threshold test. The sensing threshold is defined as the lowest sensitivity setting (i.e. the highest mV value) at which the pacemaker consistently senses intrinsic activity. Most modern pacemakers offer automatic testing options for sensing thresholds. One such option, automatic P and R wave measurement, provides values of intrinsic signals which can be evaluated to see if the sensitivity setting is programmed efficiently. Manual testing involves decreasing the pace rate to allow the intrinsic rate to break through and then confirming that intrinsic events are sensed. An annotated rhythm strip can be useful to confirm sensing (Figs 14.3 &14.4).

If necessary, the sensitivity setting may have to be adjusted to assure proper sensing. The normal sensing safety margin is half the value, i.e. if the pacemaker can sense reliably at 5.0 mV, a good setting (with safety margin) is 2.5 mV.

Step six: systematic ECG analysis

Using the paced ECG, study the ECG carefully to see how the pacemaker and patient are interacting.

Nearly every available pacemaker seen in clinical practice today offers annotated ECG strips, so clinicians have the luxury (and the reassurance) of seeing events exactly as the pacemaker interprets them. While every manufacturer uses a slightly different annotation system, most are intuitive to those familiar with pacing.

There will be letter codes identifying events, such as AS (for atrial sensed event), AP (for atrial paced event), VS (for ventricular sensed event) and VP (for ventricular paced event). Intervals are stated numerically, often with horizontal lines to help show where they belong. The advantage of annotation, besides ease of use, is that the pacemaker itself is reporting how it "sees" such events. When it senses atrial activity, it documents it in the annotations as intrinsic atrial activity.

While annotations can be useful, they must never replace the information on the actual tracing. For instance, a pacemaker may annotate events that are not there on the strip (such as oversensing) or may not annotate events that are clearly present (such as undersensing).

In order not to miss subtle problems or overlook signs of potential trouble in the ECG, it is recommended that the clinician work through the following checklist.

1 Are the programmed settings consistent with the strip?

2 Is there reliable capture, with every pacing spike leading to a depolarization?

3 Is the QRS morphology normal or does there seem to be ventricular fusion (i.e. ventricular paced and sensed events "morphing" together in an odd-shaped QRS)? Note that a notched QRS complex may be indicative of left bundle branch block. This is not a cause for reprogramming, merely of clinical awareness.

4 Is sensing appropriate? Does sensed activity inhibit an output pulse? Does sensed atrial activity result in paced (or sensed) ventricular activity?

5 Is the rhythm synchronous or are there isolated P and R waves?

6 How would you categorize the patient's underlying rhythm?

7 Does it seem from the strip that the patient might benefit from features that are available but possibly not activated in the device? Such features are described in Table 14.2.

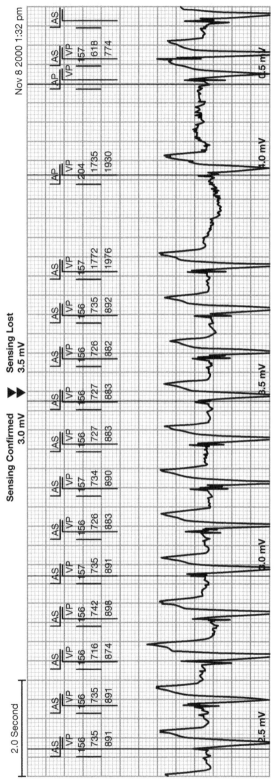

Fig. 14.3 Atrial sensitivity test in a patient with AV nodal block. Note that sensing was lost at 3.5 mV but restored at 3.0 mV.

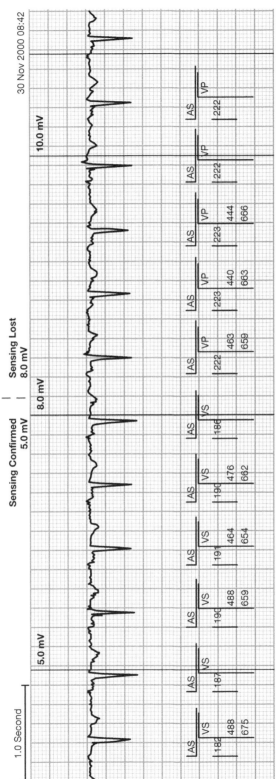

Fig. 14.4 A ventricular sensitivity test for a dual-chamber pacemaker patient with intact AV conduction. Sensing was lost at 8.0 mV but restored at 5.0 mV.

Table 14.2 Pacemaker feature assessment

Pacemaker feature	Patient might benefit from it, if he has:	Things to consider:
Mode switching	Lots of high-rate atrial activity with rapid ventricular response	Mode switch transitions can be abrupt; program a mode switch base rate if available
PMT algorithm	High intrinsic ventricular activity	This is a good feature to program on for almost any patient, even if there is no apparent PMT problem
Rate response	Patient complains that he can't exercise as much as he wants and there is an absence of chronotropic response (higher sinus rates during exercise)	Activate rate-responsive AV/PV delay values as well
AF Suppression™ algorithm	Atrial fibrillation, whether or not it conducts; if mode switching is active, there may be lots of mode switch episodes	Overdrives atrium at dynamic rate corresponding to patient's intrinsic atrial rate

Step seven: stored EGMs

An intracardiac electrogram (EGM or sometimes IEGM) is similar to a surface ECG, except the electrical signals used to create the tracing are generated from within the heart. The value of the EGM is that it shows you the ECG the exact way the pacemaker "sees" it. While reading an EGM is not very different from reading an ECG, there are subtle distinctions – such as the size of the signals – that provide additional valuable clues as to what the pacemaker is sensing in the heart.

Just as pacemakers can store numerical data in the form of event counters, which result in histograms, bar charts, trends, and other visual formats, the latest generation of pacemaker can now store a complete EGM in memory. Since IEGM storage uses a lot of memory, there is a limited capacity. For that reason, the clinician should make some decisions in advance as to what kind of EGMs would be most useful, so that the right information is put into memory.

During follow-up, the clinician may download EGMs that were generated because a "trigger" or specific precondition was met. Triggers can be high-rate activity, a PVC, or other cardiac event. EGMs may be programmed for single-channel, dual-channel, or cross-channel.

A single-channel EGM records information only from one chamber of the heart, typically the ventricle. A single-channel EGM is the only option for a single-chamber pacemaker, but dual-chamber systems may be programmed to deliver a single-chan-

nel EGM. A single-channel EGM takes up less space in memory, allowing for more and longer EGMs than the other options. If activity in one chamber is of more interest than the others or if the clinician wants to be sure to maximize EGM storage capacity, a single-chamber EGM may be the best choice.

A dual-channel EGM provides the complete picture of a dual-chamber pacing system. Clearly, it is the option that provides the clinician with the most information. On the other hand, a dual-channel EGM contains so much information that it's a memory hog! It limits the overall capacity for storing electrograms significantly. When the clinician does not anticipate triggering a lot of EGMs or does not feel the need to see a large quantity of data, the dual-channel EGM is the best choice (Fig. 14.5). It does provide the highest-quality EGM.

A recent innovation in the world of stored EGMs is the new cross-channel EGM. Available only for dual-chamber pacemakers, the cross-channel EGM blends data from both the atrial and ventricular channel to create a single stored EGM. A cross-channel EGM is a technical hybrid, of sorts, and can take some practice to be able to read. The advantage of a cross-channel EGM is that it provides the benefits of atrial and ventricular data without the need for large amounts of device memory. When good quality data in fairly large quantities are anticipated, a cross-channel EGM offers the best solution.

When doing follow-up, access the stored EGMs and review the programmed EGM triggers. Although an EGM can provide a great snapshot of how the pacemaker saw the heart at a specific point

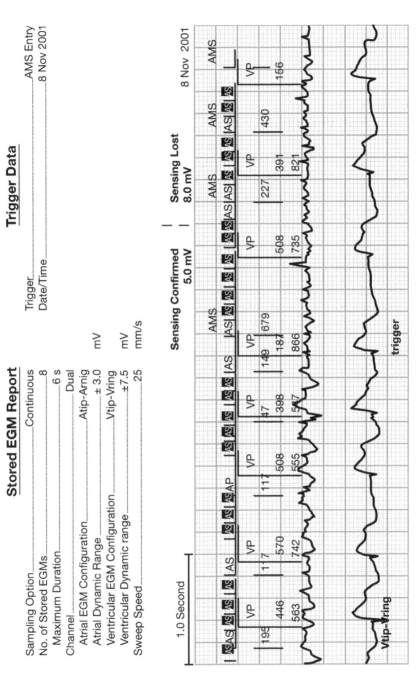

Stored EGM Report

Sampling Option	Continuous
No. of Stored EGMs	8
Maximum Duration	6 s
Channel	Dual
Atrial EGM Configuration	Atip-Aring
Atrial Dynamic Range	± 3.0 mV
Ventricular EGM Configuration	Vtip-Vring
Ventricular Dynamic range	±7.5 mV
Sweep Speed	25 mm/s

Trigger Data

Trigger	AMS Entry
Date/Time	8 Nov 2001

Fig. 14.5 Stored dual-channel EGM triggered by entry into the mode switch algorithm (AMS is noted at the top of the AS and AP annotations). The top tracing shows the atrial channel, indicating an atrial tachycardia that develops into atrial fibrillation. The lower tracing shows the ventricular channel. Note that the EGM is triggered by the AMS entry but commences the EGM with almost 3 s of data preceding the triggering event.

in time, it only "takes the picture" according to how the previous clinician programmed the pacemaker. Review the programmed settings carefully.

For this reason, the clinician conducting follow-up should give some careful consideration to programming the settings for stored electrograms for the next follow-up, which is likely to occur 6 months in the future (or more, if the patient puts it off).

Step eight: document, document, document

One of the pillars of good clinical practice has to be meticulous record keeping. The printouts obtained during the session should all go into the patient's chart. Fortunately, many manufacturers now make printing from the programmer very easy. Some programmers even print out on standard-sized paper which fits nicely into a chart folder. The running ECG, the programmed parameters as they were when the patient arrived, and printouts of stored EGMs of interest should all be included, along with the clinician's notes and observations.

One purpose of follow-up is to adjust programmable parameters as necessary to improve device performance. Carefully document any programmable settings that have been changed by printing out "before" and "after" programmed parameter pages. Most programmers will somehow flag any parameters that have been changed.

Some physicians are in the habit of printing the currently programmed parameters twice, in order to give a printout to the patient to take home. Should the patient consult other physicians or for some reason need to see a different doctor about the pacemaker (for instance, during travel or emergencies), the printed record can greatly facilitate the next consultation. For patients who are willing to keep track of these papers or those who travel a great deal, this is a recommended course of action.

Before the follow-up is concluded, diagnostic counters and memories should be cleared. This allows the device to clear its memory and reset itself for the next 6 months.

Further reading

ACC/AHA/NASPE. *Guideline Update for Implantation of Cardiac Pacemakers and Antiarrhythmia Devices*, 2002.

Bernstein AD, Irwin ME, Parsonnet V *et al.* Report of the NASPE Policy Conference on antibradycardia pacemaker follow-up: effectiveness, needs and resources. *PACE* 1994; **17**: 1714–29.

Fraser JD, Gillis AM, Irwin ME *et al.* Guidelines for pacemaker follow-up in Canada: a consensus statement of the Canadian Working Group on Cardiac Pacing. *Can J Cardiol* 2000; **16**: 355–76.

Medicare Coverage Issues Manual. Baltimore: US Dept of Health and Human Services, Health Care Financing Administration, 1990. HCFA publication 6 Thur Rev. 42.

Schoenfeld MH, Marokowitz HT. Device follow-up in the age of automaticity. *PACE* 2000; **23**: 803–6.

The nuts and bolts of systematic follow-up

- Systematic follow-up streamlines the process of follow-up while providing assurance that you do not inadvertently skip steps or overlook "hidden" problems.
- There are eight steps in systematic follow-up:
  1 patient interview
  2 running ECG
  3 download diagnostics
  4 capture threshold testing
  5 sensing threshold testing
  6 systematic ECG analysis
  7 stored EGMs
  8 document, document, document!
- Accurate record-keeping is essential for providing good patient care. When in doubt, write it out.
- Lead impedance values should be checked at each follow-up; a large, sudden change in lead impedance value is indicative of a possibly severe lead problem.
- Transtelephonic patient monitoring (TTM) is a well-proven method of obtaining basic

Continued p.129

Continued.

information from the pacemaker without requiring the patient to come into the office. There are limitations to TTM: you cannot adjust parameter settings. It offers a good alternative to the regular check-up for stable patients who become comfortable with the system.
- Many pacemakers offer one-button follow-up or other automated sequences. These features are usually worth using because they are quick and will not let you accidentally omit a step.
- It may be good practice to print out the device settings at the end of the follow-up session and give a copy to the patient to carry in his or her wallet.
- Always clear diagnostic counters at the conclusion of the follow-up session.
- Pacemaker guidelines call for dual-chamber pacemakers to be followed every 6 months, and single-chamber pacemakers to be followed annually (twice in the first 6 months post-implant, then yearly thereafter).

CHAPTER 15

Troubleshooting and diagnostics

Pacemaker diagnostics is a broad term that covers a wide variety of reports (histograms, counters, graphs, bar charts, and so on) available through the programmer. For decades, pacemakers have been able to collect data on how they operate, store it in their memory, and report it back in specialized formats to clinicians. While diagnostic data have been around for years, it is only recently that diagnostics have become relatively straightforward and easy to use. Many pacemaker diagnostic reports are readily available in the first programming steps (with no special steps for downloading) and present data in readable, intuitively clear formats. Some diagnostics even allow the clinician to select a preferred report format.

During routine follow-up, it is important to download the basic diagnostic data from the pacemaker, even if no particular problems are suspected. One benefit of checking diagnostic reports is that problems that might have otherwise been hidden (e.g. if the patient was asymptomatic or the problem did not show up on an ECG) come to light and can be addressed before they become serious issues. Most experienced pacemaker experts have turned up evidence of a dislodged lead or suboptimal device settings long before the patient realized anything was out of order.

When checking routine diagnostics for a patient with no particular complaints, it is important to address the questions in the following list.

- Are there any unexpected findings in any of the diagnostics? For example, are there relatively high numbers of mode switch episodes, premature ventricular contractions (PVCs), high rate activity?
- Is the device pacing more than one might expect?
- What pacing states are involved? For instance AP–VS pacing means that conduction is intact. AS–VP pacing indicates intrinsic atrial activity. Are the pacing states consistent with the patient's rhythm disorder?

- Are there rate variations that seem inappropriate (for instance, is there a lot of high rate pacing in a sedentary patient)?
- If the device is rate responsive, is there a reasonable amount of sensor-driven activity? Is the sensor-driven rate appropriately high (or not high enough)?
- Are there trends that indicate changes in threshold, activity levels, or the presence of atrial arrhythmias?

When checking diagnostics, download them at the outset of the programming session and print them out. Once they are safely printed, clear the diagnostics. This zeroes out the counters. Sometimes, it may be useful to check on diagnostic counts amassed during the actual follow-up session. Before the patient leaves the clinic, clear the diagnostics again. This ensures that at the next follow-up session, there will be only the latest data.

Diagnostic counters can be valuable in getting a general overview of how the patient and pacemaker are interacting, but diagnostics can be even more valuable when trying to track down a specific problem.

Today's pacemakers offer so many programmable features and settings that there has never been a time when pacing therapy could be better individualized to meet a patient's unique needs. Unfortunately, the fact that patients are unique means that it is impossible to spell out anything like a "systematic guide to troubleshooting." Troubleshooting, more than any other aspect of pacemaker patient care, involves detective work, differential diagnoses, and a thorough familiarity with device options. It can also take a certain measure of patience and perseverance.

Since troubleshooting always involves "trouble" of one sort or another, this chapter will address some of the most common problems encountered during follow-up.

The Nuts and Bolts of Cardiac Pacing, 2nd edition. By Tom Kenny. © 2008 St Jude Medical, ISBN: 978-1-4501-8403-8.

Intermittent or permanent loss of capture

Capture is the single most important thing that a pacemaker does, so when capture becomes unreliable – or is lost altogether – the patient loses all benefit of the pacing system. Loss of capture may be intermittent or permanent, and clearly can be of serious consequence for pacemaker-dependent individuals.

There are many things that can cause non-capture. In troubleshooting capture problems, the clinician has to work through the list, ruling out likely causes (Table 15.1).

- **Inappropriate output settings.** In this case, establish the capture threshold and program the appropriate safety margin.
- **Elevated threshold.** This can occur naturally over time or be the result of some change in disease progression, drug regimen, or other factor.
- **Lead problems**, including dislodgement (acute phase) or damage of some kind to the lead. Impedance values should be double-checked; a chest X-ray may be required.
- **Battery depletion** (end-of-life). Check the battery status, usually shown on the programmer screen. Older devices may require a special test sequence, often relying on a magnet. If the battery is wearing down, schedule elective replacement surgery. In the interim, modified output settings may be able to spare some battery life (providing they still offer reliable pacing therapy).
- **Component failure.** While this is very rare, it has been known to occur. It should probably be checked only after all other causes of non-capture have been ruled out. A good resource for suspected component failure is the technical services department of the manufacturer. Most manufacturers operate 24-h hotline services for questions about their products. When confronting an unusual situation, this technical service is one of the best resources.

Sensing problems

Sensing problems are probably the single most common troubleshooting topic pacing experts encounter. There are two main types of sensing problems: oversensing and undersensing. Oversensing means the device is sensing things it should not be sensing; oversensing leads to underpacing. Undersensing, on the other hand, means the pacemaker is not sensing things it ought to be sensing; undersensing leads to overpacing (Table 15.2).

Sensing problems are typically diagnosed when paced ECGs are evaluated. Sensing problems may be intermittent or more constant. For dual-chamber pacemaker patients, it is possible to have sensing problems in one chamber but not in the other. Although severe sensing problems may cause symptoms, many patients with transient sensing problems are asymptomatic.

Undersensing

Undersensing in a dual-chamber pacemaker may also reveal itself by an unusually high number of PVCs in the diagnostic counters. The pacemaker defines a PVC as two ventricular events without an

Table 15.1 Troubleshooting guide to capture problems

Questions	If ...	Then...
How old is the pacemaker system?	If it is new	The lead might be dislodged
	If it is old	Then the battery may be depleted
Is the patient on any drugs?	If there are new drugs	His threshold may have changed
	If there are several drugs	His threshold may be elevated by polypharmacy
What are lead impedance values?	If there has been a big change (>200 Ω)	There could be damage of some sort to the lead or the lead connection
	If the lead impedance is very high	The lead could be broken or not connected properly in the pacemaker header
	If the lead impedance is very low	The insulation could be compromised or torn

Table 15.2 Troubleshooting guide to sensing problems

Problem	Diagnostic toolkit	Most likely remedies
Oversensing and undersensing	Sensing threshold tests Annotated IEGM and ECG	Reprogram sensitivity setting
Non-capture	Capture threshold test Annotated IEGM and ECG	Reprogram output (pulse amplitude and/or pulse width)
Backup mode	Annotated IEGM and ECG Programmer notification	Reprogram (see manual) out of backup
Crosstalk	Annotated IEGM and ECG Oversensing	Extend ventricular blanking period; decrease ventricular sensitivity (higher mV value); decrease atrial output
Rate variations	Check programmed parameters Annotated IEGM and ECG Rate histogram	Reprogram sensitivity (device may be oversensing)

intervening atrial event. A small number of PVCs is normal for most patients and some patients may be particularly susceptible to them. For a dual-chamber pacemaker patient with intrinsic atrial activity, a high PVC count could signal that not all atrial activity is being properly counted – and that means atrial undersensing.

The potential causes of undersensing include:
- inappropriate programming
- lead dislodgement (acute phase)
- connector problem (more likely in acute phase)
- lead damage (insulation breach or lead fracture)
- component failure.

Usually undersensing can be addressed by reprogramming the sensitivity setting to a lower mV value (i.e. making the device more sensitive). If a lower mV setting seems to be the best solution to undersensing, be careful not to overcompensate and make the device overly sensitive (leading to oversensing). In fact, overcompensation on sensitivity settings may be one of the main causes for oversensing and undersensing. Unfortunately, there is no universal formula to arrive at the right sensitivity setting for every patient, and sensitivity settings often need to be adjusted for the same patient over time, so it is good strategy to check sensitivity thresholds during every follow-up session.

Oversensing

Oversensing can appear on the ECG or EGM as long pauses or "missed beats." The pacemaker does not seem to be pacing as much as it ought to. An annotated strip can confirm oversensing by showing where the pacemaker has noted a sensed event that does not show up on the tracing itself.

Diagnostic counters give evidence of oversensing by offering a lower-than-anticipated percentage of paced events or cardiac activity at a rate lower than the programmed base rate (or hysteresis rate, if programmed). Oversensing means that the pacemaker is inhibited when it ought to be pacing; an inhibited pacemaker relies on the patient's escape rhythm to take over. Since the escape rhythm is probably much slower than the programmed base rate, diagnostics may uncover periods of below-base-rate cardiac activity. This is a classic diagnostic "clue" that oversensing is going on. The patient may be asymptomatic, particularly if the oversensing is brief or intermittent.

The main causes of oversensing are given in the following list.
- **Inappropriate programming**: the sensitivity setting may be so sensitive that it is detecting signals that are not really there. To decrease sensitivity, *increase the mV setting*. Sensitivity settings may require adjustments over time, so they should be checked at every follow-up. When making changes to the sensitivity setting, be careful not to overcompensate. Making the pacemaker too insensitive will cause undersensing!
- **Crosstalk**: which occurs when the ventricular lead misinterprets an atrial output pulse as an intrinsic ventricular event. Crosstalk does not occur in all patients and depends, to some degree, on variables beyond the clinician's immediate control: the patient's anatomy, lead placement,

and energy requirements of the atrial output setting. Pacemakers may offer specific parameters to minimize crosstalk; even older models can be programmed to reduce crosstalk by extending the ventricular refractory period.

- **Myopotentials** or muscle noise that is inappropriately interpreted by the pacemaker as intrinsic activity. Bipolar leads are less susceptible to myopotentials than unipolar leads, but lead revision (in the event unipolar leads are in place) is a major step. The first attempt at managing this situation is decreasing the device's sensitivity to filter out myopotentials while still allowing sensing of appropriate cardiac signals. Many physicians prefer to implant a bipolar system initially to avoid this problem altogether.
- **Electromagnetic interference (EMI)**: the world is full of electromagnetic signals, some of which can affect pacemakers. When patients have ongoing problems with EMI, oversensing will be reported in the diagnostic data (or possibly on stored electrograms) but not during real-time ECGs taken at follow-up. An audit of the patient's activity may be required to determine the source of the EMI. Sometimes, the best course of action is to provide the patient with information about EMI sources and how to handle them.
- **Polarization potentials**: this is residual energy or noise in or around the heart. Polarization potentials cannot be reduced or avoided; if they occur, the device must "program around" them by either reducing sensitivity (i.e. increasing the mV setting) or by extending the appropriate blanking periods to "cover up" the period when polarization potentials occur.
- **Lead dislodgement (acute phase)**: lead problems can sometimes manifest as sensing problems. This is more likely during the period immediately after implant. Once a pacemaker has demonstrated reliable sensing, a sudden episode of oversensing is unlikely to be caused by a lead problem.

Interference (backup pacing mode)

Most pacemakers offer backup pacing options which occur automatically when certain conditions are met (such as running into EMI). It is possible to see a patient in follow-up with a pacemaker in a backup mode, typically asynchronous pacing. Since asynchronous pacing is not pleasant for most patients, these patients will usually report symptoms. A pacemaker can usually be readily programmed out of the backup pacing mode with a few simple programming steps. It may be necessary to consult the device manual.

Pacemakers should not go into backup mode except under "extreme" circumstances, such as prolonged exposure to EMI or some other type of problem, even component malfunction. Thus, it is important not only to restore normal pacing operation, but to determine why the pacemaker reverted to backup mode in the first place. If the patient remembers unusual events or could feel when the pacemaker changed operation, this may provide insight into why the backup occurred. One of the most likely reasons for backup reversion is EMI.

A patient in backup mode because of EMI requires basic information about the nature of EMI, potential sources of EMI, and strategies for managing electromagnetic fields in his environment. It is impossible to say with certainty that any general category of appliance or tool is or is not a source of EMI (e.g. some drills may be a source of EMI that affects the pacemaker, while other drills may not be). In addition, people may be exposed to "hidden" EMI when they shop in large stores (theft detection systems). Everyday life involves exposure to EMI when people travel (airport screening systems) or enter public buildings (metal detectors).

Should backup reversion because of EMI become a chronic problem for a particular patient, it is worthwhile discussing the situation with the device manufacturer. A field clinical engineer may be able to work with the patient in his own environment to help measure and assess EMI sources.

Rate variations

Variations in the pacing rate may be a source of concern for both patient and clinician. In very advanced and well-programmed systems, there may be a multiplicity of variables that influence the pacing rate, including hysteresis rate, sensor-driven rate, maximum tracking rate, maximum sensor rate, and rest rate. As such, the more advanced and carefully programmed the system, the less likely you are to see a clockwork-like ECG of pacing all at one constant rate. The healthy human heart beats at different rates over the course of a day, and the well-paced heart mimics that behavior. Nevertheless, rate alterations can be a cause of symptoms and concerns in the patient.

As a rule of thumb, diagnostic data should reveal heart rates that fall into categories appropriate for the patient's lifestyle. A bedridden or wheelchair-bound patient should exhibit lower rates overall than an exuberant pediatric patient. Wide swings in rates are only appropriate for patients who lead very active lifestyles. A preponderance of high-rate activity is probably not appropriate for any patient.

On the other hand, most pacemakers today have numerous parameters that can impact on the rate. The old days of Earl Bakken's first metronome-like pacemaker are over! When troubleshooting rate variations, these programmable features and parameters and how they impact the rhythm strip need to be considered:

- rate response should increase the rate during periods of exercise
- AF Suppression™ should overdrive the atrium at a rate slightly above the intrinsic rate and allow for ventricular tracking in response
- rest rate will decrease the rate to a programmable rest rate during profound inactivity or sleep
- hysteresis will allow the intrinsic rate to prevail even when it is slightly below the base rate (check the programmable hysteresis rate)
- there may be ceilings established on certain rates: maximum tracking rate or maximum sensor rate set upper rate limits for the system.

However, there may be variations in rate which cannot be attributed to programmable features. In some cases, rate variations may occur because of:

- programmed settings that are not appropriate for the patient (e.g. overly aggressive rate response, a very low maximum tracking rate (MTR), very low hysteresis values, a high base rate, and so on)
- backup mode can force pacing at a fixed rate
- end-of-life of the device can force fixed-rate pacing
- oversensing (the device underpaces and thus the rate is lower)
- component malfunction (very rare).

In the very early days of pacing, it was sometimes possible in clinical practice to see a pacemaker pacing constantly at a very high rate. This condition – colorfully described as "pacemaker runaway" – has been almost completely eradicated in the past two decades by the application of a special circuit which prohibits pacing above a certain rate under any circumstances.

When troubleshooting rate problems, the first step is to check that programmed parameters which affect the rate are appropriate for the patient. Check rate response (sensor settings, maximum sensor rates), hysteresis rate, maximum tracking rate, and the base rate. Since pacemaker patients may be seen – and reprogrammed – by other clinicians, there is no guarantee that even your own patients will return to follow-up programmed to the last settings you selected. Many rate problems can be solved simply by adjusting the programmed settings to more appropriate values.

Advanced settings

Some of the newest features promoted by the various manufacturers actually arose from the common troubleshooting issues in clinical practice. For example, high-rate atrial activity was met by the introduction of mode switching. If a patient regularly experiences high atrial rates with rapid ventricular response, mode switching can effectively "turn off" the atrial channel so the ventricle cannot respond to it.

Atrial fibrillation – once even a contraindication for a dual-chamber pacemaker – posed clinical problems, so that the AF Suppression™ algorithm and other overdrive algorithms were introduced. For patients plagued by atrial fibrillation, these algorithms allow the pacemaker to overdrive (and thus control) the atrium.

For patients with pacemaker-mediated tachycardias, PMT options allow these to be automatically addressed. Matching diagnostic features provide counts of PMT events for the clinician.

The AutoCapture™ pacing system not only addresses intermittent loss of capture through normal threshold variations, it reduces the amount of energy the device needs by eliminating the need to program a conventional (2:1) safety margin.

When possible, it is recommended that clinicians take advantage of these sophisticated features, most of which can be programmed in one or two simple, intuitive steps. These features were created to simplify pacing therapy or address common problems.

When older pacemakers need replacement, one of the best arguments for getting sophisticated new technology is that it solves so many of the old troubleshooting problems.

Further reading

Ellenbogen KA. *Cardiac Pacing*, 2nd edn. Cambridge: Blackwell, 1996.

Geppert A, Rauscha F. Pacemaker dysfunction in clinical practice. *Wien Klin Wochenschr* 2001; **113**: 15–26.

Hayes DL, Vliestra RE. Pacemaker malfunction. *Ann Intern Med* 1993; **119**: 828–35.

Okreglicki A, Akiyama T, Ocampo C *et al.* Polarization potentials causing pacemaker oversensing. *Jpn Circ J* 1998; **62**: 868–70.

Paraskevaidis S, Mochlas S, Hadjimiltadis S *et al.* Intermittent P-wave sensing in a patient with a DDD pacemaker. *PACE* 1999; **22** (4 Part 1): 689–90.

The nuts and bolts of troubleshooting

- The main causes of intermittent or permanent loss of capture are an inappropriate output setting, an elevated pacing threshold, trouble with the leads, or battery depletion.
- Oversensing means the same thing as underpacing (i.e. not pacing when the pacemaker ought to pace). Likewise, undersensing means the same thing as overpacing (i.e. pacing when it is not necessary or appropriate).
- The main causes of undersensing problems are inappropriate programming and lead problems. In the acute phase, undersensing might be caused by lead dislodgement or a connector problem.
- Sensitivity settings (in mV) affect how the pacemaker senses. The lower the mV value, the more sensitive the pacemaker. Thus, if a pacemaker is undersensing, make sure the sensitivity is high enough (i.e. decrease the mV value).
- The main causes of oversensing are inappropriate programming and various types of interference, including crosstalk, myopotentials, EMI and polarization potentials. Lead dislodgement may occur in the acute phase.
- Crosstalk occurs when the ventricular lead inappropriately senses the atrial output and interprets it as intrinsic ventricular activity.
- There are many potential sources of EMI which can cause problems for a pacemaker, even causing it to go into backup mode. Patients may require education about EMI sources and how to avoid them.
- Backup mode may occur for several reasons, and it is important to understand why the device reverted to backup mode. Most pacemakers can be quickly and easily programmed out of backup mode with a few simple programming steps.
- Component failure is extremely rare in pacemakers today, but if it should occur, it might manifest itself as capture or sensing problems.
- Rate variations are most likely caused by inappropriately programmed parameter settings. There are many parameters that impact rate, which should be checked.
- Manufacturers operate a technical services department to help troubleshoot difficult or unusual cases. They should be consulted when routine tactics fail to get to the root of specific problems.

CHAPTER 16

Advanced features

Pacemakers have a long-standing tradition of continuing innovation, and nowhere is that innovation more evident than in the sophisticated special features designed to address the needs of certain pacemaker patients. Special features describe the functionality that is generally available in most current products and which is appropriate for many, if not most, pacemaker patients. Advanced features are those special capabilities that are either not available in all current products on the market or that may not be suitable for a wide range of patients.

The decision to use special and advanced features is always one of clinical judgment, based on the patient's needs, underlying rhythms and other conditions. Downloadable diagnostics provide an opportunity at follow-up sessions to check how the patient and pacemaker have interacted with these special features.

AutoCapture™ pacing systems

Capture is fundamental to any pacing system, but the amount of energy required to capture the heart is a value that fluctuates over the course of a day and over time. It is well accepted that immediately following implantation and for several weeks thereafter, the pacing system goes through an acute to chronic threshold change. The implantation of the pacing electrode causes an inflammatory process to occur at the myocardial interface that creates an increase in the capture threshold. After a few weeks, the capture threshold returns to normal and stabilizes. Unfortunately, in many patients the capture threshold may vary owing to other conditions, such as electrolyte imbalance, acid–base imbalance, drug therapy and heart failure. In addition, everyday activities such as exercise, eating and even sleeping can alter the pacing threshold. These dynamic changes in capture threshold are a threat to the safety of the patient because they are often unpredictable. Most

clinicians program a generous safety margin or "extra energy" to ensure that the pacemaker system delivers more than enough energy in every output pulse to capture the heart. Although a generous safety margin ensures reliable capture, it also wastes energy, which could lead to premature depletion of the battery.

The AutoCapture™ pacing system was designed to ensure reliable capture on a beat-by-beat basis without the need for a large safety margin. To accomplish this, the AutoCapture™ algorithm assesses the threshold on every beat and adjusts the pacing output values accordingly. It also confirms capture every beat. If an output does not capture the heart, a backup pulse is delivered to make sure that the heart is paced at the appropriate rate. The theory behind AutoCapture™ pacing systems is that if capture thresholds can be assessed at every beat, far less energy will be needed to operate the system, particularly over the long term. With capture confirmation, the AutoCapture™ pacing system is safer than a conventional system (even one with a large safety margin) because capture is assessed for each beat (Fig. 16.1).

The AutoCapture™ algorithm relies on the evoked response (ER) as well as "residual polarization" to function. The theory is that a pacemaker output of sufficient energy will cause the heart to depolarize (i.e. capture). The ER is the signal that indicates that the heart is responding to this output by depolarizing at the myocardial level; the residual polarization (sometimes just called "polarization") is an electrical phenomenon that occurs owing to the delivery of the pacing pulse regardless of capture. In other words, polarization occurs after pacing. Knowing the difference between an ER and residual polarization is what allows the AutoCapture™ algorithm to distinguish whether a pacemaker spike caused depolarization or not. When capture is confirmed, the

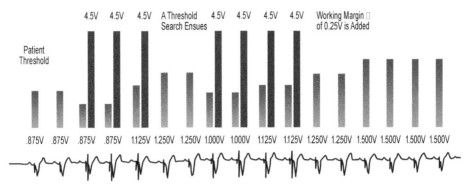

Fig. 16.1 AutoCapture™ pacing systems provide beat-by-beat capture confirmation. A working safety margin of 0.25 V is added to each output pulse. The light grey bars show capture. When capture did not occur, a backup safety pulse of 4.5 V was delivered (dark grey bar) and the pacing output pulse adjusted upward.

algorithm measures the capture threshold and self-programs the output settings so that the next output pulse will be 0.25 V above the measured capture threshold (working margin). In the event that capture is not confirmed, a 4.5 V backup pulse is delivered for safety (Figs 16.2 & 16.3).

Although AutoCapture™ pacing is automatic, it requires some special testing both at implant and periodically during follow-up to work at optimum levels. The test measures the ER and the polarization signal amplitudes. A clinician is required to initiate the test, carried out on the programmer, and then wait until it completes on its own. During the test, the AV and PV delay are temporarily programmed to 25 and 50 ms, respectively, so that ventricular pacing is forced. While ventricular pacing is going on, the system measures the amplitude of the ER and the amplitude of the residual polarization signal. During the test, the programmer will prompt the clinician to program a setting for the ER sensitivity level. The programmer will automatically recommend an appropriate value, which the clinician can accept or override by programming a new

value. The test completes when ER and polarization signals are measured.

At this point, the clinician should initiate the AutoCapture™ pacing systems threshold test. This is another automatic test that is simply programmed to start and then allowed to complete automatically. In the test, the AV and PV delays are temporarily programmed to 25 ms and 50 ms, respectively, again to force ventricular pacing. The output is then stepped down in 0.25 V increments until capture is lost. (For patient safety, any loss of capture is handled by the 4.5 V backup pulse.) When two output pulses at the same value fail to capture the heart, the system calls this the sub-threshold value. Starting with the sub-threshold value, the output pulse is now increased in 0.125 V increments until capture is restored. The point at which capture is restored is called the threshold value. The pacemaker then automatically programs itself to deliver an output pulse 0.25 V above the determined threshold value. This margin (known as the "working margin") is just to "round up" the value for better efficacy. It should not be thought of in the same way as the "safety margin."

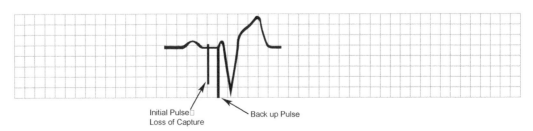

Fig. 16.2 Capture is determined by detecting an evoked response (ER) from the lead tip on every single beat. If there is no ER, a backup safety pulse of 4.5 V and 0.5 ms is delivered.

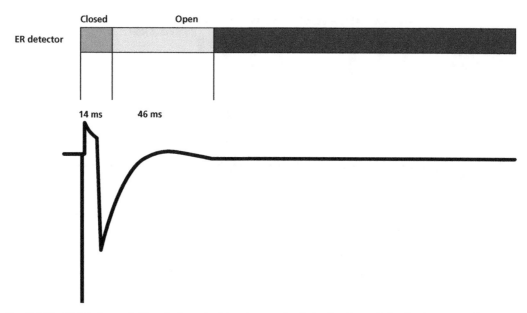

Fig. 16.3 The ER detector works like a timing cycle; it is not responsive during the 14 ms window it takes to pace the ventricle. After that, it "opens" and is alert to possible signals.

In fact, if the safety margin has any counterpart in the AutoCapture™ pacing system, it would be in the form of the 4.5 V backup pulse.

One distinction between the AutoCapture™ pacing system and other pacemakers with similar functionality is that the AutoCapture™ algorithm checks and verifies capture on each and every beat. Other systems verify capture much less often, sometimes only as frequently as once every few hours.

When capture is lost, the backup pulse is delivered and a threshold search ensues. The threshold search is an automatic function that increases the output pulse amplitude until capture is restored (Figs 16.4 & 16.5).

When capture is lost, the AV/PV delay is automatically extended by 100 ms on the next beat. This extension, called the "fusion avoidance algorithm" or FAA, was created to minimize fusion-induced threshold searches. A fusion beat occurs when a pacemaker output and an intrinsic beat collide; on the ECG it looks like a particularly large or emphatic paced beat. This event can prompt the AutoCapture™ pacing systems to search for a new threshold. By extending the AV and PV delay following a backup safety pulse, this is often avoided (Fig. 16.6).

By monitoring capture and adjusting the pacing output accordingly, a pacemaker with the AutoCapture™ system uses significantly less energy than a comparable system programmed with the old safety margin. In fact, it is not unusual to see projected 100% pacing longevity projections of 10 years or more for AutoCapture™ pacing systems. This has also allowed for radical downsizing of full-featured pacemakers.

Currently, AutoCapture™ pacing systems are only available on the ventricular channel. The first pacemakers with the AutoCapture™ algorithm only had a unipolar backup safety pulse. Today, the 4.5 V backup safety pulse can be programmed to a bipolar or unipolar configuration, depending on physician preference.

It is generally agreed that pacing thresholds change in an individual over time. This has posed a real clinical challenge, because it is not clearly understood when and how they change in any particular patient. It is well accepted that non-capture occurs in 1–5% of pacemaker patients at any given time, but it has been difficult to say in which patients and at what times. For this reason, clinicians have accepted the safety margin – a deliberate waste of energy – to ensure the most critical function of the pacemaker, namely capture. Using the diagnostic in an AutoCapture™ pacing systems device allows physicians to look back and see just how often pac-

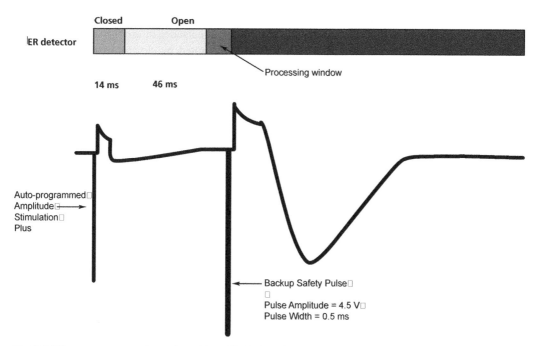

Fig. 16.4 When capture cannot be confirmed by an ER, the AutoCapture™ pacing systems deliver a backup safety pulse.

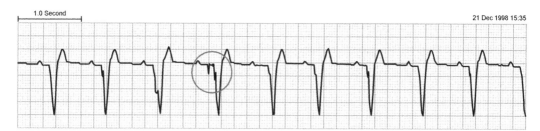

Fig. 16.5 On an ECG, an initial output pulse appears but fails to capture the ventricle. This is promptly followed by the backup safety pulse.

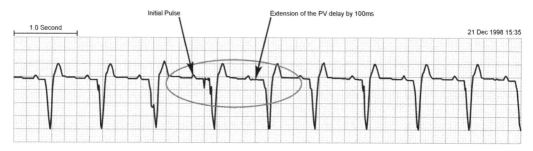

Fig. 16.6 A backup safety pulse is delivered and the next PV delay (which starts with the sensed atrial event in the circle) is automatically extended by 100 ms. This helps to prevent the next ventricular pacing spike from landing on an intrinsic beat and prompting a threshold search.

ing thresholds actually change. The present-generation devices have the ability to store diagnostics of threshold values at various measurement points as well as during adjustments. Such information can be very useful in assessing a patient's condition and guiding future programming decisions.

The key to the AutoCapture™ system is that it monitors and adapts the pacing output on a beat-by-beat basis to maintain maximum safety with minimal output. In other words, *it delivers only the output that is needed* to maintain capture on every single beat. In this way, it uses energy more efficiently without sacrificing the most important pacemaker function, capture.

The reasons for using AutoCapture™ pacing systems in patients are:
- capture confirmation on every beat with a backup safety pulse in the event of non-capture enhances patient safety by assuring that capture occurs
- AutoCapture can respond to fluctuations and even major changes in the capture threshold
- by using less energy over the long term, it may preserve battery life and thus extend device longevity.

AF Suppression™ algorithm

Atrial fibrillation is the single most common arrhythmia in the world and its prevalence increases with age. In the early years of pacemakers, atrial fibrillation was actually a contraindication to dual-chamber pacing and it remains a confounding variable in finding the ideal pacing prescription. Pacemakers with mode switching algorithms can "turn off the atrial channel" during episodes of high atrial rate activity, but that only addresses how the device deals with an ongoing arrhythmia – it does not address the arrhythmia itself.

Long spells of atrial tachycardia or atrial fibrillation reduce a dual-chamber pacemaker patient to a patient who has a functional single-chamber pacemaker! There is also evidence that atrial fibrillation worsens over time and is associated with an increased risk of stroke. The phrase, "A-fib begets A-fib" describes how the vicious cycle of atrial fibrillation can perpetuate. The more you keep the atrium and ventricle in synchrony with each other, the fewer arrhythmias a patient will have.

The AF Suppression™ algorithm was designed to suppress episodes of atrial fibrillation. It had long been noted by electrophysiologists that it was possible to "overdrive" the atrium by pacing it slightly faster than the native rhythm. The paced outputs captured and controlled the atrium and prevented the native rate from taking over. If the overdrive commenced before the atrial activity became very rapid, the patient could have an atrial overdrive rate that controlled the atrium at a high but manageable rate. The benefit of atrial overdrive was that it suppressed atrial fibrillation, i.e. the overdrive algorithm never allowed atrial fibrillation to start.

An overdrive rate can control the atrial rate as well as the rhythm. It works by minimizing ectopic beats, long–short cycles, and dispersion of refractoriness. By overdriving the atrium and imposing a slightly fast but regular rhythm, the atria do not lapse into fibrillation.

Early atrial overdrive algorithms were simply high atrial-paced rates. There was one significant problem with these original algorithms: to be high enough to overdrive the atrium, they had to be fairly high. Pacing at such high rates was often uncomfortable for the patient.

The AF Suppression™ algorithm was shown to be clinically effective in the ADOPT-A clinical trial. It works on the same principle as the atrial overdrive algorithm, except that the overdrive rate the atrium uses is dynamic and based on the patient's own intrinsic rate. The algorithm works by monitoring the patient's atrial rate and then adapting the AF Suppression™ rate to a rate slightly above the intrinsic rhythm. This preserves a high percentage of atrial pacing. In fact, studies have shown that the AF Suppression™ algorithm generally allows 90% atrial pacing.

The advantage of using a dynamic atrial overdrive algorithm is that it is adapted to the patient's own rate. If the patient is active, the overdrive rate is higher than it would be when the patient is at rest. In all cases, it is high enough to overdrive the atrium (Fig. 16.7).

The pacemaker is always looking at a 16-cycle window. When the pacemaker finds two intrinsic atrial events (P waves) in this window, then the AF Suppression™ algorithm automatically increases

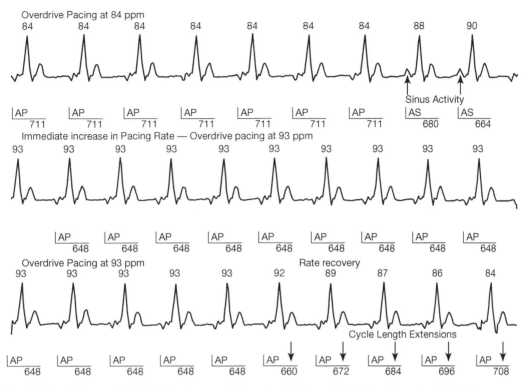

Fig. 16.7 The AF Suppression™ algorithm shows overdrive pacing at 84 ppm, which is then interrupted by intrinsic sinus activity at an even higher rate. This prompts an immediate increase in the atrial pacing rate, forcing the system to overdrive the atrium at 93 ppm After a programmed number of cycles at this overdrive rate, the pacemaker gradually lengthens cycles to search for intrinsic activity and reduce the rate. These changes are automatic and are based on the patient's own prevailing rate (which could be paced, sensor-driven, or intrinsic).

the atrial pacing rate between 5 and 10 bpm (the actual increment depends on the patient's paced rate at that moment). The atrial stimulation at the higher rate is delivered for a programmable number of overdrive cycles. Should two intrinsic P waves be detected before the programmed number of overdrive cycles is completed, then the atrial paced rate is increased automatically.

Once the programmed number of overdrive cycles has been delivered, the atrial pacing rate is decreased according to a programmable rate recovery sequence. Basically, cycle lengths are extended gradually until the applicable pacing rate (which is either base rate, rest rate or sensor-indicated rate) is reached.

The design of this algorithm avoids prolonged periods of high-rate atrial pacing and it will not activate if there is no intrinsic high-rate atrial activity nor will it activate when the sensor is controlling a higher atrial rate.

The AF Suppression™ algorithm can be an important feature for patients who have or might develop atrial fibrillation. As many people fall into this category, it might seem that the AF Suppression™ algorithm is right for everybody. There are, however, patients for whom it is not appropriate.

• The AF Suppression™ algorithm was designed to suppress episodes of paroxysmal and persistent atrial fibrillation; it was not designed to address permanent atrial fibrillation.

• Patients may develop atrial fibrillation suddenly, even if they had no indication of it previously. The incidence of atrial fibrillation increases with age and disease progression. Thus, many pacemaker patients who do not have atrial fibrillation today may be expected to develop it in the future. The AF Suppression™ algorithm is a good safety net.

• The AF Suppression™ algorithm is *not* useful for patients who have complete heart block, AV nodal ablation, or silent atria.

During follow-up, it is useful to check the AT/AF burden trend and related diagnostic reports, including an AF Suppression™ histogram, to evaluate how the algorithm is working for a particular patient. This histogram shows the rate distribution of atrial activity driven by the AF Suppression™ algorithm along with the total percentage of atrial paced events and the percentage of time spent in mode switching.

Controlling atrial fibrillation can be very important to pacemaker patients.

- Atrial fibrillation can interfere with AV synchrony and cause uncomfortable and even debilitating symptoms.
- "AF begets AF" means that once atrial fibrillation starts, it tends to keep going and get worse. Suppressing atrial fibrillation can stop the vicious cycle.
- Atrial fibrillation is typically treated with drugs; if the AF Suppression™ algorithm can suppress it, the patient may be spared having to take one more drug.
- Unlike cardiac drugs, the AF Suppression™ algorithm is not compromised by patient compliance issues. When programmed on, it works constantly in the background without requiring the patient's compliance. Patients may not even be aware of it.
- The ADOPT-A study showed that patients treated with the AF Suppression™ algorithm had no side-effects from it.
- The AF Suppression™ algorithm could potentially reduce the number of painful cardioversions for some patients.

Rate-Responsive PVARP/VREF

Many things can affect the pacing rate of a dual-chamber pacemaker: intrinsic activity, sensor control, rest rate or other algorithms. The pacing rate affects all of the dual-chamber timing cycles, including the PVARP and VREF cycles. The Rate-Responsive PVARP/VREF feature automatically increases or decreases the refractory period interval appropriately as the rate changes. Without this special feature, most clinicians program a relatively low maximum tracking rate (MTR), above which the pacemaker cannot pace the ventricle. This works relatively well in patients who do not require higher

pacing rates. It keeps the values of PVARP and VREF timing cycles within fairly limited values. But what about patients who might benefit from an occasional higher MTR value? These are patients who might like to exercise or who lead very active lives. Programming a higher MTR did not work well for them because the PVARP and VREF values would not allow pacing above a certain rate.

The Rate-Responsive PVARP/VREF values can be programmed to high, medium, low or off. Each value imposes an algorithm. For example, when programmed to medium, the algorithm decreases the PVARP value by 2 ms per ppm change in the patient's rate. For example, a patient's intrinsic rate increases by 5 bpm, which means the PVARP value would decrease by 10 ms (5 × 2 ms). If the PVARP had been programmed to a setting of 275 ms, the new automatically shortened PVARP value would now be 265 (275 – 10) (Table 16.1).

This special feature is only active when the patient's rate is 90 ppm or higher. As the algorithm adjusts the timing cycles, it attempts to maintain a 25 ms spread between the PVARP and the VREF. If the PVARP is set to a value 25 ms above the VREF, then PVARP shortens until it is 25 ms greater than the VREF setting. Thereafter, both PVARP and VREF will decrease together and maintain the 25 ms spread. If the difference between PVARP and VREF is < 25 ms, then both values change concurrently. Rate-Responsive PVARP/VREF continues to shorten refractory periods until the interval reaches the programmed "Shortest PVARP/VREF" parameter setting.

The Shortest PVARP/VREF parameter allows the clinician to program the shortest time allowable for the PVARP and VREF when Rate-Responsive PVARP/VREF is enabled. The settings are 120–230 ms in steps of 10. The nominal value is 200 ms.

Table 16.1 Rate-Responsive PVARP/VREF settings

Rate-Responsive PVARP/VREF setting	Rate of shortening
Off	0
Low	1 ms per bpm/ppm
Medium	2 ms per bpm/ppm
High	3 ms per bpm/ppm

This feature is available for most modes, including single-chamber (AAIR and VVIR) as well as dual-chamber (DDDR, DDIR, VDDR, DVIR).

Although Rate-Responsive PVARP/VREF may seem like a complicated or limited feature, it can be a very valuable feature when the clinician wants to allow a patient to have a particularly high maximum tracking rate (MTR) without compromising overall device performance. In addition, this feature allows a longer sensing window, which can reduce or eliminate competitive pacing (pacing into intrinsic activity). Shorter refractory periods mean more atrial activity gets sensed, which in turn could mean that the mode switch algorithm goes into effect sooner during periods of rapid intrinsic activity.

Who can benefit from Rate-Responsive PVARP/ VREF?:

- patients who rely on mode switching for high-rate atrial activity
- patients who could benefit from a higher than usual MTR (active, athletic patients in particular)
- patients who have or might experience competitive pacing.

Programmable Absolute Atrial Refractory Period

This special feature only applies to atrial single-chamber pacing, so it may seem to have limited utility. Although atrial single-chamber pacemakers are not common, this feature allows the clinician to blank far-field R waves to get better sensing in the AAI and AAIR modes (as well as AAT, AATR, OAO, and OAOR modes).

An atrial event – either paced (A) or sensed (P) – launches a refractory period, which consists of two parts. There is an absolute atrial refractory period (during which nothing is sensed) followed by a relative refractory period (during which sensing occurs but the pacemaker classifies anything it senses as "noise" and may launch its noise response). The pacemaker is not alert to sense atrial events until the relative refractory period is over.

This feature allows the clinician to program the absolute atrial refractory period. The total atrial refractory timing cycle (programmable absolute atrial refractory plus the relative atrial refractory period) remains the same, but the proportion of time that is "absolute" versus the "relative" time changes. The value of this feature resides in the fact that sometimes atrial pacemakers pick up ventricular activity (known as "far R" or "far-field R waves") and inappropriately classify it as noise (causing the pacemaker to revert to noise response) or inappropriately sense it (causing the pacemaker to count it as a sensed atrial event). By programming the absolute period to be long enough to "cover" the anticipated ventricular activity, it is possible to find an elegant programming solution to this problem (Fig. 16.8).

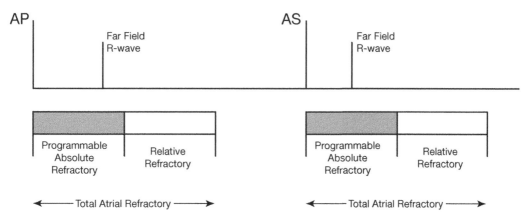

Fig. 16.8 The total atrial refractory period is composed of an absolute refractory period followed by a relative refractory period. The ability to extend the absolute segment of the atrial refractory period allows the clinician to control the atrial activity the pacemaker "counts" and responds to.

This feature is important when trying to optimize programming in a single-chamber atrial system, particularly when there is the possibility of far-field R wave sensing.

Negative AV Hysteresis with Search

Hysteresis with search (discussed earlier) encourages the patient's intrinsic rate to prevail; for most patients, that is the best course of treatment. Certain patients, however, may benefit more from paced than intrinsic activity, and that is when the opposite feature, Negative AV Hysteresis with Search, can be used. Negative AV Hysteresis *encourages the device to pace the ventricle*. This feature can be useful if the patient's hemodynamics benefit from consistent pacing. One indication for Negative AV Hysteresis with Search is the patient being paced for hypertrophic obstructive cardiomyopathy or HOCM. Another application would be in biventricular pacing, during which the hemodynamic benefits are obtained by forcing pacing to bring the ventricles back into better synchrony.

Negative AV Hysteresis works by programming a negative or offset value, typically about –40 ms. The Negative AV Hysteresis goes into effect with any atrial event, either sensed (P wave) or paced

(A). If an intrinsic ventricular event is sensed during the normal sensed or paced AV delay timing cycle, then the pacemaker automatically shortens the programmed sensed or paced AV delay by the programmed offset, in this case, by 30 ms. Thus, if a sensed ventricular event occurs during the paced AV delay and the paced AV delay has been programmed to 150 ms, this advanced feature automatically shortens the paced AV delay to 110 ms (150 – 40 = 110). This automatic shortening encourages ventricular pacing (Fig. 16.9).

When programming Negative AV Hysteresis, it is also important to program a value for the shortest allowable sensed or paced AV delay. This sets a minimum value below which the pacemaker will not go. By programming an appropriate minimum sensed or paced AV interval, proper timing of the atrial and ventricular activity can be assured.

Like regular hysteresis, Negative AV Hysteresis has a search function, during which the sensed or paced AV interval is extended to allow the pacemaker to "search" for intrinsic activity.

Negative AV Hysteresis is not a clinically relevant feature for the majority of pacemaker patients, as most pacemaker patients derive greater benefit from more intrinsic activity than from more paced activity. For those instances when it is important to

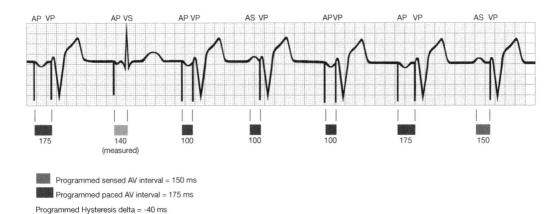

Fig. 16.9 In this strip, Negative AV Hysteresis is programmed on. The sensed AV delay is 150 ms and the paced AV delay is 175 ms. A hysteresis delta of –40 ms is programmed. Negative AV Hysteresis works by shortening the paced or sensed AV delay to force pacing.

encourage long-term ventricular pacing, however, this feature can be extremely valuable.

Ventricular Intrinsic Preference™ Technology

The Ventricular Intrinsic Preference (VIP)™ algorithm was designed to allow the pacemaker to search periodically for intrinsic ventricular activity and to adjust the sensed or paced AV delay in order to encourage intrinsic activity over right-ventricular pacing. In dual-chamber modes, the VIP algorithm searches for intrinsic conduction, adjusting the sensed or paced AV delay in such a way to encourage to the native ventricular event to inhibit pacing. This algorithm promotes intrinsic conduction (when possible) and helps minimize unnecessary right-ventricular pacing, both of which are thought to benefit the patient.

The clinician first programs a search cycle, which is programmable in time (every so many minutes) and by cycle (number of cardiac cycles). During the search intervals, the algorithm automatically extends the length of the programmed sensed or paced AV delay in an effort to see if any intrinsic ventricular events will break through. The amount by which the sensed or paced AV delay is extended is programmable. The search interval searches for the total number of cycles programmed. (For example, if you program to extend the sensed or paced AV delay by 160 ms for three cycles and search every 5 minutes, then every 5 minutes the AV delay will be extended by 160 ms for three cycles. If an intrinsic ventricular event occurs in one of those three cycles, the extended AV delay remains in effect until three cycles with no intrinsic ventricular activity are counted.)

A Cap Confirm

Pacemakers are becoming increasingly automatic since many of the housekeeping checks that were typically performed by clinicians can actually be done by the device itself. A new pacemaker now offers automatic atrial capture verification. This feature, called A Cap Confirm™, automatically adjusts the atrial pulse amplitude in response to the patient's activity.

It has a programmable search function, during which time it overdrives (force-paces) the atrium. It then verifies capture by stepping down the atrial pulse amplitude in small (0.25 V) steps until three consecutive beats occur at loss of capture.

When loss of capture occurs, the device is set up to automatically deliver a 5.0 V backup pulse. In this way, the patient continues to receive the benefits of atrial pacing even during the capture verification process.

Once capture is lost in three consecutive beats, the atrial pulse amplitude is then slowly incremented (0.125 V steps) until there are two consecutive paced atrial events. These two-step protocols (one step-down, the second step-up) proceed automatically with no clinical intervention.

A Cap Confirm can be programmed on or off, but it may also be set to monitor. In monitor mode, A Cap Confirm observes atrial activity and reports to the programmer how it would have performed had it been activated. In this way, a clinician can "test-drive" the function before actually programming it on.

Further reading

Binner L, Messenger J, Sperzel J et al. AutoCapture enhancements. *PACE* 2003; **26** (1 Part 2): 221–4.

Carlson MD, Ip J, Messenger J et al. A new pacemaker algorithm for the treatment of atrial fibrillation: results of the Atrial Dynamic Overdrive Pacing Trial (ADOPT). *J Am Coll Cardiol* 2003; **42**: 627–33.

Danilovic D, Ohm OJ. Pacing threshold trends and variability in modern tined leads assessed using high-resolution automatic measurements. *PACE* 1999; **22** (4 Part 1): 567–87.

Erdinler I, Akyol A, Okmen E et al. Long-term follow-up of pacemakers with an AutoCapture pacing system. *Jpn Heart J* 2002; **43**: 631–41.

Orem RC, Ahmad S, Siudyla P. A novel approach to the management of symptomatic, junctional and ectopic rhythms. *J Interv Cardiac Electrophysiol* 2003; **9**: 353–6.

The nuts and bolts of advanced features

- Advanced features are features that are available only in certain specific devices or features with a clinical utility for a smaller number of patients.
- AutoCapture™ pacing systems promote patient safety by assuring beat-by-beat confirmation of capture and pacing with a backup safety pulse in the event of non-capture. In this way, AutoCapture™ pacing systems can dispense with the standard 2:1 or 3:1 safety margin and use less battery energy to pace the patient reliably.
- AutoCapture™ works automatically by checking an evoked response or ER, which is the heart's natural response to capture.
- The AF Suppression™ algorithm is a dynamic atrial overdrive algorithm that was designed to suppress atrial fibrillation.
- Atrial fibrillation is the number one arrhythmia in America and is associated with numerous risk factors, including increased risk of stroke.
- The AF Suppression™ algorithm works automatically by detecting rapid atrial activity and then overdriving the atrium at a rate slightly above (5–10 ppm) the patient's intrinsic rate.
- Although exact statistics are unknown, many pacemaker patients have atrial fibrillation at implant, and many more develop it as their heart disease progresses.
- Rate-Responsive PVARP and VREF allows for these timing cycles to shorten as the pacing rate increases, while maintaining a proper relationship to each other (the system tries to preserve a 25 ms spread) and staying within programmed limits. The advantage of a rate-responsive PVARP and VREF is that it gives clinicians more flexibility to program higher maximum tracking rates without compromising pacing efficacy.
- Rate-Responsive PVARP and VREF can also be useful to help fight competitive pacing, which occurs when the pacemaker paces into intrinsic activity. (This occurs when intrinsic activity falls into the PVARP or VREF and ends up not being counted; by shortening the PVARP and VREF, more intrinsic activity is sensed and properly counted.)
- The Programmable Absolute Atrial Refractory Period is only used in single-chamber atrial systems. It prevents far-field sensing of ventricular activity, which the pacemaker sometimes inappropriately "recognizes" as intrinsic atrial activity.
- Negative AV Hysteresis is the opposite of regular AV Hysteresis, in that regular hysteresis promotes intrinsic activity while negative hysteresis promotes ventricular pacing.
- Ventricular Intrinsic Preference™ technology was designed to encourage native ventricular activity to inhibit right-ventricular pacing. It does this by extending the sensed or paced AV delay during programmable search functions to allow any intrinsic ventricular events to prevail.
- A Cap Confirm can automatically verify and provide atrial capture in advanced pacemaker systems.

Chapter 17

Clinical trials on pacing

So much device knowledge has come to us in recent years from clinical trials using implantable cardioverter-defibrillators and cardiac resynchronization therapy devices that is may be hard to believe there are comparatively few pacemaker clinical studies. During the early years of pacing, clinical trials were not as common as they have become in our own era of evidence-based medicine. Besides that, clinical trials using devices pose special problems. To accomplish a blinded study, all patients must be implanted with the same devices although devices may be programmed differently; this can make a device trial very expensive, particularly if a thousand or more patients are desired. When all patients get a device that can be easily reprogrammed, studies tend to have more drop-outs than in studies where changing therapy involves more elaborate steps. Further, programming variations may be necessary for individual patients, but can sometimes impact results.

Most of what we know about pacing has come to us from experience with the millions of pacemaker patients around the world. But, as is often the case, sometimes cherished assumptions have been challenged by clinical trials. This recently happened in pacing with the so-called DAVID study. At first glance, the DAVID study (**D**ual-Chamber **a**nd **V**VI **I**mplantable **D**efibrillator Trial) seems like it has nothing to do with pacing. The DAVID investigators implanted the patient population (n=506) with implantable cardioverter defibrillators (ICDs)! But it was what DAVID found out about pacing in these ICDs that surprised even many pacing veterans.

It is important to note some of the background of the DAVID trial, which began enrolling patients in October of 2000 and was published on Christmas Day, 2002. ICDs were increasingly being implanted both for standard indications and for primary prevention. Most ICDs have full-featured pacing

functionality. The question was whether standard-indication ICD patients who did not have a pacing indication would benefit from cardiac pacing. All DAVID patients had a conventional ICD indication but were excluded if they had a standard indication for a pacemaker.

DAVID patients had to have a left-ventricular ejection fraction of 40 percent or below (meaning they had some degree of compromised systolic function), a standard ICD indication, and they could not have a standard pacing indication or frequent uncontrolled episodes of atrial tachyarrhythmias. All DAVID patients received pharmacological therapy for their heart disease (about half were taking ACE inhibitors and beta-blockers).

The thinking behind DAVID was that dual-chamber or "physiologic" pacing might offer benefits to patients that single-chamber pacing did not. The belief was that dual-chamber pacing decreased the chances of atrial tachyarrhythmias, which might, in turn, reduce the risk of stroke. In fact, investigators wondered if turning on dual-chamber pacing might even confer a mortality as well as a morbidity benefit on patients.

Furthermore, maintaining a relatively rapid pacing rate would boost cardiac output, which, in turn, would improve overall hemodynamics.

Thus, the study was devised in such a way that all patients received an ICD but patients were randomized into two groups: one group was paced at 70 ppm in DDDR mode, while the other group received so-called "back-up pacing," that is pacing only at 40 ppm in VVI mode (Fig. 17.1.) Patients were followed at 3, 6, and 12 months, with the primary endpoint death for any reason or first hospitalization for worsening congestive heart failure. This was a composite endpoint, meaning either criterion would satisfy the endpoint. The results were unexpected (Fig. 17.2).

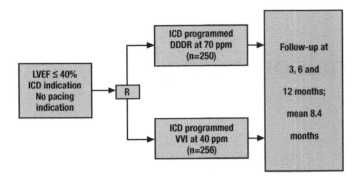

Fig. 17.1 The DAVID study was a large, randomized, controlled clinical trial.

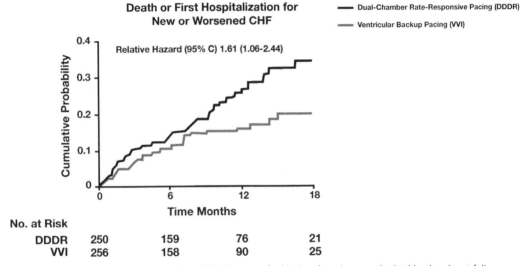

Fig. 17.2 The DDDR-70 group had a significantly higher rate of achieving the primary endpoint (death or heart faliure-related hospitalization) compared to the VVI-40 group.

Not only was dual-chamber pacing at 70 ppm not helping patients, it appeared to be harmful (Fig. 17.3). So what was really going on? While many experts were quick to say right-ventricular (RV) pacing is harmful, I am not sure that this is the real story.

The two groups in DAVID were described at DDDR-70 and VVI-40 but it would be more accurate to call them the "paced group" and the "unpaced group." A follow-up article published by Dr. Bruce Wilkoff (the principal investigator of the DAVID trial) reported that pacing occurred more than 50% of the time in the DDDR-70 group but never more than 3% of the time in the VVI-40 group. The study was not so much about pacing modes (DDDR vs. VVI) as about RV pacing versus non-RV pacing. So why was receiving a lot of RV pacing so detrimental in these patients with some degree of left-ventricular (systolic) dysfunction?

First, let's look at how a pacing works. Dual-chamber pacing from the right atrial appendage involves stimulating the right atrium and allowing the

1 year event rate	Combined	CHF	Death
VVI-40	16.1%	13.3%	6.5%
DDDR-70	26.7%	22.6%	22.6%
P-value	0.03	0.07	0.15

Fig. 17.3 DAVID found that greater amounts of RV pacing were associated with increased morbidity (CHF hospitalization) and mortality.

impulse to conduct outward over the left atrium and also downward to the AV node and ventricles. This inter-atrial conduction time (the time it takes for an impulse to travel from one atrium to the other) is longer than normal. It's artificial. Furthermore, as the impulse conducts down to the ventricles, it also imposes an artificial AV delay, even if the atrial output pulse conducts normally to the ventricles. What this means is that the normal cardiac pumping sequence (passive filling of the ventricles, atrial contraction and contribution to ventricular filling, followed by ventricular contraction) may no longer match up precisely with the electrical sequence (atrial output pulse, electrical energy delivered to the ventricles to force a contraction). Last but not least, pacemakers pace the right ventricle. In the healthy unpaced heart, electrical conduction flows downward from the right atrium, more evenly over the right and left ventricles. If ventricular pacing occurs, the energy is delivered near the bottom of the right ventricle (apex) and must travel outward and upward. This creates an artificial ventricular activation.

All of these things together may be thought of as inducing a form of pacemaker-mediated ventricular dyssynchrony. The pumping action of the heart is no longer precisely in sync with the electrical activity going on. Not allowing enough time for adequate ventricular filling (even just by a split second) can have significant hemodynamic consequences. So why were these negative aspects to RV pacing never observed before? It is my opinion that in patients with good left-ventricular function, that is, relatively normal systolic and diastolic function, RV pacing can be well tolerated. The human heart has compensatory mechanisms that can make up for the small degree of mechanical dyssynchrony than RV pacing induces.

But remember, DAVID patients were not only not indicated for pacing, they had some LV dysfunction to begin with. In fact, the median left-ventricular ejection fraction (LVEF) of the patients was 28% (VVI-40 group) and 26% (DDDR-70 group). These patients had ventricular dysfunction and the introduction of RV pacing just exacerbated the condition.

The VVI-40 group was paced so little that they did not experience the same impact from pacing. Before we get too far along, it is important to remember there DAVID does not explore the now very intriguing question: do ICD patients with LV dysfunction *and a standard bradycardia pacing indication* derive benefit from pacing or not? We just do not know.

The most important take-away message from DAVID is that *unnecessary RV pacing should be avoided*, particularly in patients with compromised LV function. But was the problem just RV pacing in and of itself? Many pacing veterans (including me) think that AV timing may be the real culprit. Pacing imposes artificial timing cycles on the heart, which govern its pumping function according to precisely timed electrical events. Allowing an artificial AV delay to take control of the heart's pumping function can adversely affect hemodynamics.

New work to better time or optimize the AV delay holds out some promise for this condition. Imaging techniques (notably with echocardiography) have been used to help visualize the interaction between pacing cycles (electricity) and pumping cycles (mechanics). St. Jude Medical ICDs with dual-chamber pacing offer a device-based algorithm called the QuickOpt™ algorithm to accomplish AV timing optimization in a simple programming step, in a way that correlates very closely with echocardiographic results.

But what was the role of RV pacing? The DAVID II study results were announced in 2007. This study compared AAI-70 pacing to VVI-40 back-up pacing in the same type of pacing (LVEF ≤ 40%, standard ICD indication, no pacing indication). The use of the AAI mode at 70 ppm assured that the patients would be paced often but that RV pacing was impossible. At 28 months of follow-up, it was announced that there was no significant difference between groups for such endpoints as death, hospitalization for heart failure, or the occurrence of atrial fibrillation. This seems to further indicate that unnecessary RV pacing should be minimized in such patients. But the reason why is unclear: is it RV pacing in and of itself or could it have something to do with the AV delay timing? Neither DAVID trial optimized AV delay timing. The real answer may be that it is more important to optimize the AV interval than to prevent RV pacing.

As a result of the DAVID study, many physicians became more judicious in their use of RV pacing. Manufacturers have developed new pacemaker features (which can be found in pacemakers as well as ICDs) to reduce unnecessary RV pacing. However, the real mechanisms behind the DAVID study results remain elusive.

A few months before the DAVID trial was published, the MOST study results were published. MOST stands for **Mo**de **S**election **T**rial in Sinus-Node Dysfunction. A total of 1,014 patients with sinus node dysfunction and, thus, a standard pacing indication were randomized to receive either dual-chamber or single-chamber pacing. The objective was to compare mortality rates, heart failure hospitalizations, incidence of atrial fibrillation (AF), and the occurrence of pacemaker syndrome and some other functional characteristics. Overall, dual-chamber patients did better. Dual-chamber pacing reduced the risk of AF, reduced signs and symptoms of heart failure, and improved quality of life. However, dual-chamber pacing did not improve stroke-free survival when compared to single-chamber pacing.

The MOST trial is probably most important for what it did not find. All patients in MOST were exposed to what might be called "conventional RV pacing." Yet there were no deleterious effects reported. Neither group reported worsening heart failure. In fact, heart failure scores improved with DDD pacing compared to VVI pacing. How can we harmonize the MOST results with the DAVID findings? MOST patients were indicated for pacing! As for LV dysfunction, the MOST study does not report median LVEF scores at baseline but does indicate that over 80% of the MOST patient population had New York Heart Association Class I or Class II heart failure at baseline (the least severe forms). Surely, a subset of the MOST patients would have likely had some degree of LV dysfunction, but the study did not specifically address that.

One thing the MOST study investigated was so-called "pacemaker syndrome." This is a constellation of signs and symptoms associated with single-chamber pacing. The MOST study had a very large number of patients in the single-chamber group cross over to the dual-chamber group. It is possible that the cross-over rate was so high in MOST because cross-overs were permitted and relatively easy. However, it is clear from the MOST study at least that many patients prefer dual-chamber pacing for the simple reason that it makes them feel better. Most pacing physicians have observed this same phenomenon anecdotally.

The CTOPP study, which stands for the Canadian Trial of Physiological Pacing, was first published in 2000 and then extended study results were published in 2004. This study enrolled patients indicated for conventional pacing for symptomatic bradycardia (that is, for sinus node dysfunction or heart block or both) and compared ventricular single-chamber pacing to dual-chamber "physiologic" pacing. Neither the first or extended study found any mortality benefits to dual-chamber pacing compared to single-chamber pacing, but the extended study reported a persistent significant reduction in the development of AF with dual-chamber pacing.

Clinicians still have a strong preference for dual-chamber pacing, and some of this is fueled by their own anecdotal observations of the reactions of patients on VVI versus DDD pacing. It remains to be determined whether "pacemaker syndrome" will ever be measured in a meaningful way in a clinical trial. When it comes to things like morbidity and mortality, dual-chamber pacing does not offer an overwhelming advantage over single-chamber pacing. While we have no hard data that dual-chamber pacing confers significant clinical benefits over single-chamber pacing in many patients indicated for pacing, most clinicians believe that dual-chamber pacing is the better choice. They usually point out things like this:

- Dual-chamber pacing is designed to deliver one-to-one AV synchrony, which would assure sound hemodynamics
- Dual-chamber pacing has been shown to reduce atrial tachyarrhythmias
- If the patient does not have heart block, dual-chamber pacing can assure ventricular rate support without RV pacing

Thus, clinicians have naturally put these clinical trials into perspective, that is, they are valuable information but are only tools to assist in the complicated real-world practice of cardiac pacing. Patients are complicated and there is value in putting experience as well as evidence to work in their care.

RV pacing is clearly something that should not be used indiscriminately, especially in patients with systolic dysfunction. The role of AV timing in physiologic pacing requires further exploration, since it may play a very important role in optimal pacing therapy. While there is no clinical evidence that physiologic (dual-chamber) pacing confers mor-

tality benefits over single-chamber pacing, there is clinical evidence that dual-chamber pacing reduces atrial tachyarrhythmias and anecdotal support that many pacemaker patients prefer it. Based on what we know today, the best way to approach pacing includes these steps:
- Pace only patients who have a standard indication for bradycardia pacing
- Program the pacemaker appropriately, including AV delay, rate, and the use of algorithms to minimize unnecessary pacing
- Follow the patient regularly and review and adjust pacing parameter settings as needed

To be sure, there is still a lot we have to learn about the electrical management of cardiac rhythm disorders. But it is important that we put clinical evidence to practical application, and that requires good clinical judgment. We know that millions of people have benefited from cardiac pacing and millions more will continue to do so in the future. The DAVID trial and other studies should not make us fearful, it should make us prudent. The attitude one sometimes hears about avoiding RV pacing altogether is an extremist position that throws the baby out with the bathwater. When it comes to conventional pacing, follow-up care should not be about minimizing RV pacing at any cost; it should be about optimizing AV intervals.

Further reading

Connolly SJ, Kerr CR, Gent M et al. Effects of Physiologic Pacing versus Ventricular Pacing on the Risk of Stroke and Death due to Cardiovascular Causes. *N Engl J Med* 2000; **342**: 1385–91.

Kerr CR, Connolly SJ, Abdollah H et al. Canadian Trial of Physiological Pacing: Effects of Physiological Pacing During Long-Term Follow-Up. *Circulation* 2004; **109**: 357–62.

Lamas GA, Lee KL, Sweeney MO et al. Ventricular Pacing or Dual-Chamber Pacing for Sinus-Node Dysfunction. *N Engl J Med* 2002; **346**: 1854–62.

Tang AS, Roberts RS, Kerr C et al. Relationship between Pacemaker Dependency and the Effect of Pacing Mode on Cardiovascular Outcomes. *Circulation* 2001; **103**: 3081–5.

The DAVID Trial Investigators. Dual-Chamber Pacing or Ventricular Backup Pacing in Patients with an Implantable Defibrillator. *JAMA* 2002; **288**: 3115–23.

Wilkoff BL and the DAVID Investigators. The Dual-Chamber and VVI Implantable Defibrillator (DAVID) Trial: Rationale, Design, Results, Clinical Implications, and Lessons for Future Trials. *Card Electrophysiol R* 2003; **7**: 468–72.

The nuts and bolts of clinical trials on pacing

- The most important pacing study to date is DAVID, which was actually a study using ICDs. DAVID suggests that RV pacing may be harmful in patients with systolic dysfunction not indicated for pacing.
- It is not scientifically sound to extend the meaning of the DAVID study beyond the actual study. DAVID did not find that RV pacing was harmful, period; it found it was harmful to patients with LV dysfunction who were not indicated for pacing.
- The DAVID trial compared DDDR pacing at 70 ppm to VVI pacing at 40 ppm. The result was it compared frequent dual-chamber pacing to very little pacing.
- It is believed that RV pacing induces a slight form of mechanical dyssynchrony which is much less well tolerated in patients with LV dysfunction than in those with more normal systolic function. It has been suggested (but not proven) that AV timing may play a role in this induced dyssynchrony.
- AV timing refers to the time between the atrial event (output pulse) and the ensuing ventricular event (paced or sensed). In the healthy heart, the AV delay allows for optimal ventricular filling time. In a paced heart, an AV delay that is "off timing" by even a split second can affect filling time.
- The DAVID II study found that AAI pacing at 70 ppm was not worse than VVI back-up pacing at 40 ppm; in other words, the negative effects of DDDR-70 pacing did not occur when AAI pacing was used. This further suggests that unnecessary RV pacing should be avoided.

Continued p.152

Continued.

- The MOST study looked at patients with sinus node dysfunction (and a conventional pacing indication) and compared single-chamber to dual-chamber modes. There was no stroke-free survival benefit to dual-chamber pacing versus single-chamber pacing, but dual-chamber pacing was associated with some benefits. Dual-chamber pacing reduced the risk of atrial fibrillation, improved signs and symptoms of heart failure, and improved quality of life.
- The CTOPP study enrolled patients with symptomatic bradycardia (and a conventional pacing indication) in a single-chamber group to a dual-chamber group. A short-range study (published in 2000) found no significant benefits to dual-chamber pacing, but an extended study (published in 2004) found that dual-chamber pacing was associated with a significantly reduced development rate of atrial fibrillation.
- Most pacing experts have observed "pacemaker syndrome," a constellation of symptoms, including malaise, associated with single-chamber pacing. Although MOST found no mortality benefits to dual-chamber pacing over single-chamber pacing, MOST did have a high rate of patients in the single-chamber group who asked to cross over to the dual-chamber group.
- To apply current clinical evidence to the practice of cardiac pacing, clinicians should pace only patients indicated for cardiac pacing, program devices appropriately, and follow them regularly, adjusting programmable parameter settings as required. The real-world practice of cardiac pacing is always a bit more complicated than what results from clinical trials would have us think!
- It's not about minimizing RV pacing, it's about optimizing AV timing!

APPENDIX

A short guide to systematic pacemaker follow-up

Although most device manuals and clinicians talk about pacemaker in terms of rate, i.e. pulses per minute (ppm), the pacemaker and programmer usually report rate as pacing intervals in milliseconds (ms). The formula for converting rate to intervals or ppm to milliseconds is 60 000/ppm = 1 ms. In other words, a pacemaker set to a base rate of 60 ppm will have pacing intervals of 1000 ms. The conversion chart in Fig. A.1 translates rate to intervals and vice versa.

When dealing with a single-chamber pacemaker, follow these steps for systematic follow-up (Fig. A.2).

1 Collect information (free-running ECG, magnet ECG, interrogation, programmed settings).

2 On the non-magnet ECG, measure the automatic/pacing interval in milliseconds. Convert it to pulses per minute.

3 Verify capture from the strip by determining each pacemaker spike lead to depolarization. Look for unusual waveform morphologies (such as wide or bizarre QRS complexes, resembling a PVC or LBBB) and see if there is any fusion. If any pacemaker spike does not lead to QRS complex, ask if it had opportunity to capture. In other words, where does the spike fall in relationship to the intrinsic refractory period? You would not expect a spike falling into this period to capture. This is called **functional non-capture,** meaning you would not expect the spike to capture.

4 Verify sensing from the strip by determining if intrinsic cardiac activities cause the device to become inhibited. Another way to assess sensing is to ask the question: does the intrinsic QRS cause the device to re-time the escape interval?

5 Assess the patient's underlying rhythm.

6 Document, document, document.

When dealing with a dual-chamber device, here are

CONVERSION CHART

ppm	ms
30	2000
35	1714
40	1500
45	1333
50	1200
52	1154
54	1111
56	1071
58	1034
60	1000
62	968
64	938
66	909
68	882
70	857
72	833
74	811
76	789
78	769
80	750
82	732
84	714
86	698
88	682
90	667
92	652
94	638
96	625
98	612
100	600
110	545
120	500
130	462
140	429
150	400
160	375
170	353
180	333
190	315
200	300

Fig. A.1 Conversion chart.

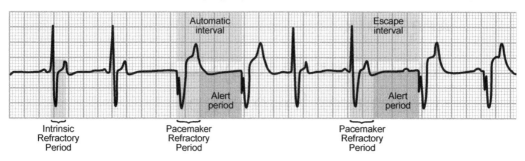

Fig. A.2 Single-chamber ECG.

the basic steps for systematic follow-up up (Fig. A.3).

1 Collect information (free-running ECG, magnet ECG, interrogation, programmed settings).

2 On the non-magnet ECG, measure the V–A or the A–A interval in milliseconds. Convert it to pulses per minute.

3 Measure the sensed and paced AV intervals.

4 Evaluate atrial capture. It is very common that the P wave caused by atrial capture will be difficult to see on the surface ECG. Look for atrial spikes followed consistently (at a normal AS–VS interval) by narrow QRS conduction. In the absence of high-grade AV block, this may be the best way to assess atrial capture.

Paced AV Interval: (AP → VP)
Sensed AV Interval: (AS → VP)
MTR: Maximum Tracking Rate
PVARP: Post ventricular atrial refractory period
VRP: Ventricular refractory period
TARP: Sensed/Paced AVD + PVARP = TARP,
        Total atrial refractory period
URL: Upper Rate Limit

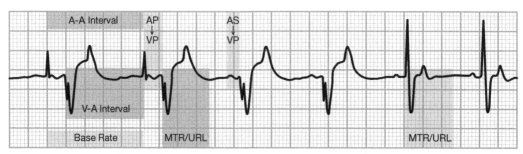

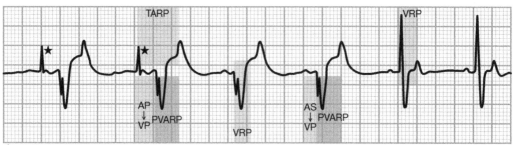

★ = V-Blanking Period

Fig. A.3 Dual-chamber ECG.

5 Evaluate ventricular capture. Evidence of ventricular capture is wide or unusual-looking QRS complexes following a ventricular pacing spike or ventricular fusion.

6 Evaluate atrial sensing by determining if intrinsic P waves are followed by ventricular pacing. If the pacemaker has ventricular timing, measure forward from a ventricular event using the VP–AP interval (base rate minus AV delay). When a P wave occurs outside the total atrial refractory period (TARP), it should inhibit the atrial output (no atrial spike). If the pacemaker has atrial timing, measure forward from an atrial event using the AA interval. Again, verify if a P wave occurring outside the TARP inhibits the atrial output.

7 Evaluate ventricular sensing. For pacemakers with ventricular-based timing, measure from a ventricular event to determine if an intrinsic ventricular event during this period inhibits the next atrial and ventricular pacemaker output. Another way to evaluate ventricular sensing (and this works for pacemakers with either ventricular or atrial timing) is to find an atrial event and measure the programmed paced AV interval. If a QRS falls in this interval, ventricular sensing is present if it inhibits the next ventricular output.

8 Assess the patient's underlying rhythm and evaluate level of pacemaker dependency.

9 Document, document, document.

Glossary

accelerometer A type of activity sensor used in rate-responsive pacemakers which detects motion along a geometric plane.

action potential The sequence of five phases (phase 0 to 4) during which cardiac cells depolarize, repolarize and then resume resting membrane potential.

active-fixation mechanism A lead with a fixation mechanism on the distal end that works by direct attachment into the endocardium. The most common active-fixation lead has an extendable–retractable screw or helix.

acute-to-chronic threshold change The observed behavior of the stimulation threshold from implant to about 8 weeks post-implant which characteristically begins low, trends sharply upward at around the second to fourth week and then decreases slightly and levels off at about 8 weeks. Large acute-to-chronic threshold changes are associated with older-generation leads and non-steroid-eluting leads. Steroid-eluting leads and even non-steroid-eluting late-generation leads do not exhibit such marked shifts in acute to chronic thresholds.

alert period In pacemaker timing cycles, the time during which the pacemaker can see and will respond to intrinsic signals. Dual-chamber pacemakers have alert periods on each channel, that is, atrial alert periods and ventricular alert periods.

algorithm A specially designed form of pacemaker behavior intended to achieve a specific goal. For example, the AF Suppression™ algorithm is a special form of dynamic atrial overdrive pacing that is designed to suppress atrial fibrillation.

anode The positive pole in any electrical circuit.

asynchronous pacing A type of pacing (VOO, AOO, DOO) in which the pacemaker paces but does not sense. This results in properly timed output pulses that are delivered, regardless of any intrinsic activity going on. Asynchronous pacing modes are rarely used except in specific test or limited situations.

atrial contribution to ventricular filling The period in every cardiac cycle when the ventricles are relaxed and the atria contract, squeezing the blood in the upper chambers into the ventricles, forcing the ventricles to stretch to accommodate this extra quantity of blood.

atrial kick A popular slang term for the atrial contribution to ventricular filling.

atrial diastole The relaxation of the heart's upper chambers.

atrial systole The contraction of the heart's upper chambers. This contraction forces the blood in the atrium into the ventricle.

atrioventricular (AV) node A group of highly specialized cardiac cells located on the right side of the interatrial septum near the opening of the coronary sinus; electrical energy collects at the AV node but gets delayed slightly, allowing for a properly timed ventricular contraction.

atrium The two upper, smaller, thin-walled chambers of the heart (plural: atria).

Auto Rest Rate. A type of pacemaker response designed to mimic the normal physiologic rate slowdown during sleep or profound rest.

automaticity The property of certain cardiac cells (particularly but not exclusively those of the SA node) that allows them to spontaneously generate electricity.

AV block A general term for many types of cardiac rhythm disorders in which the electrical impulses originating from the SA node get delayed (or sometimes entirely blocked) at the AV node. There are three degrees of AV block, with first degree the least serious. Also called heart block.

AV delay The timing cycle in a dual-chamber pacemaker initiated by a paced atrial event. If the AV delay times out before an intrinsic ventricular event is sensed, the pacemaker will deliver a ventricular output pulse.

AV synchrony The state in which there is 1:1 correspondence between atrial and ventricular activity. Patients get the greatest benefit from 1:1 AV synchrony.

base rate The rate (stated in pulses per minute or ppm) at which the clinician programs the pacemaker to pace. Typical base rate settings are 60 to 80 ppm. Sometimes called a **lower rate limit.**

bifascicular block A conduction disorder in which hemiblock (a conduction block in the left anterior or left posterior bundle branch) occurs in the setting of right bundle branch block.

bipolar Any pacing lead which has two electrodes on the distal end of the lead or any pulse generator which can accommodate such leads.

biventricular pacing Pacing and sensing both the right and left ventricles. Biventricular pacing requires a special type of device, frequently called a cardiac resynchronization therapy (CRT) device.

blind subclavian stick See Seldinger technique.

BPG British Pacing Group, an organization instrumental in developing and updating the pacemaker code.

brady-tachy syndrome A rhythm disorder in which the heart alternately beats too slowly (bradycardia) or too quickly (tachycardia). Pacing may be of special benefit in such situations, since the physician can treat the tachycardia without worrying about worsening the bradycardia component of the disorder. Sometimes called **tachy-brady syndrome.**

bradycardia Any number of heart rhythms in which the heart beats slowly. Bradycardia in athletes may be appropriate, but most bradycardias do not provide adequate rate support for daily life. A bradycardia may be chronic or intermittent and it may not necessarily cause symptoms.

can A common slang term for a pulse generator casing.

capture The occurrence of cardiac depolarization in response to an output pulse.

capture threshold. See **pacing threshold.**

cathode The negative pole in any electrical circuit.

chronaxie The point on the strength–duration curve where twice the rheobase voltage value meets the curve; this is generally the innermost portion of the curve of the strength–duration graph. The chronaxie is generally considered a reliable safety margin.

class I pacing indication Condition for which there is evidence and/or general agreement that pacing is beneficial, useful, and effective.

class II pacing indication Condition for which there is conflicting evidence and/or a divergence of opinion about the usefulness/efficacy of pacing. In class IIa, the weight of evidence is in favor of pacing, while in class IIb, usefulness and efficacy are less well established.

class III pacing indication Condition for which there is evidence and/or general agreement that pacing is not useful/effective and, in some cases, may be harmful.

coaxial lead A type of bipolar lead in which one conductor was wrapped around another conductor.

complete heart block Third-degree heart (AV) block.

conduction disorders A broad general term for conditions that can occur when the electrical system of the heart does not work properly. Arrhythmias are conduction disorders.

conduction system cells. Specialized electrical cells in the heart that allow the electrical energy produced in the heart to flow properly through the heart.

connector 1. The clear epoxy top portion of the pacemaker, into which one or more leads plugs. This is also known as the **header.** 2. The portion of the lead that plugs into the connector.

contractility A special property of myocardial cells that allows them to shorten and then return to their original length. This property allows them to stretch and then "snap back" to their original shape.

DBS A drawn brazed strand, a type of conductor wire created by a special metallurgy technique that involves drawing the wire through silver.

depolarization A cardiac contraction caused by a cellular response in which cell's change polarization (electrical) value. Individual cardiac cells depolarize and a contraction of the heart can also be described as a depolarization.

dual-chamber pacemaker A pacemaker which senses and paces in both the right atrium and right ventricle of the heart. A dual-chamber pacemaker has two leads (one for the atrium, one for the ventricle).

electrocardiogram (ECG or EKG) An electrical tracing taken from electricity measured on the surface of the skin. ECGs are commonly used to assess cardiac activity in unpaced patients. Pacemaker patients also have IEGMs from their pacemakers, which are more commonly used by their physicians to assess pacing activity.

electromagnetic interference The state that occurs when an electromagnetic field generates sufficient energy to influence pacemakers or other implanted devices. Frequently abbreviated EMI.

electrophysiologist (EP) A medical doctor who specializes in the electrophysiology of the heart and, as such, is an expert at the electrical management of cardiac rhythm disorders (pacemakers and ICDs).

electrophysiology study (EPS) Any of a series of tests on a patient conducted in an electrophysiology lab by an electrophysiologist to examine electrical conduction and possible rhythm abnormalities of the heart.

Elgiloy® The trade name for a special metallic alloy widely used in many industrial applications, including the electrodes on pacing leads.

escape interval In pacemaker timing cycles, the time from one sensed or paced event to the next sensed or paced event in that same chamber.

escape rhythm The generation of an electrical impulse by a part of the heart other than the sinoatrial (SA) node. Escape rhythms may originate in the ventricles and occur at a much slower rate than the rate that would occur if a healthy SA node was pacing the heart.

extendable–retractable lead A type of active-fixation lead in which a corkscrew-like fixation mechanism is enclosed entirely within the distal end of the lead until the point at which the physician wishes to fixate the lead; using any of a variety of methods (turning the lead, using a special tool), the corkscrew can be extended out of the lead body and fixated into the heart. Should the lead require repositioning during surgery, the corkscrew can be retracted and redeployed at another site.

fascicular block A rhythm disorder that occurs when there is a block or delay of the electrical signal in either the left anterior or left posterior fascicle of the left bundle branch. When both fascicles are affected, the condition is left bundle branch block.

fast sodium channels Special outlets in cardiac cells that allow sodium to enter or exit quickly, allowing for the rapid conduction of electrical energy and, thus, depolarization.

filar A strand of wire used in the conductor in a lead. Some leads are unifilar (one strand) while others may be multifilar (many strands).

fixation mechanism Arrangement on the distal end of a lead which allows it attach to the heart. Typical fixation mechanisms are tines (passive-fixation leads) and helices (active-fixation leads).

French A unit of measure for diameter, typically used when identifying the sizes of leads or introducers.

gap junction A special material sandwiched between cardiac cells that allows for the rapid passage of electrical energy between cells; also called intercalated disks.

header A common slang term for the clear epoxy connector top on the pulse generator, into which one or more leads plugs.

heart block A general term for many types of cardiac rhythm disorders in which the electrical impulses originating from the SA node get delayed (or sometimes entirely blocked) at the AV node. There are three degrees of heart block, with first degree the least serious. Also called AV block.

hemiblock A conduction disorder in which either the left anterior or left posterior bundle branches are blocked (fascicular block).

histogram A chart available from pacemaker programmers which depicts numerical (count) data in graphic format. One common histogram shows heart rates grouped by ranges and displayed in a bar chart.

housekeeping current The amount of energy a pulse generator consumes even when it is not in use (including before the pulse generator is implanted).

HRS Heart Rhythm Society, formerly known as the North American Society of Pacing and Electrophysiology (NASPE), an organization that advocates and promotes advanced treatment for cardiac rhythm disorders.

hybrid A small circuit board inside the pacemaker on which a variety of circuits, components, chips, and sometimes other devices (such as an accelerometer) are glued in place.

hypersensitive carotid sinus syndrome An extreme reflex response to carotid sinus stimulation which can cause syncope or presyncope in susceptible patients. Hypersensitive carotid response is defined as carotid massage that provokes asystole of three or more seconds due to sinus arrest or AV block, a substantial and symptomatic decrease in systolic blood pressure, or both.

hysteresis A programmable parameter in most pacemakers that establishes the rate at which the pacemaker will be inhibited, when that particular rate differs from the programmed base rate. For example, a pacemaker can be programmed to a base rate of 70 and a hysteresis rate of 60. That means the pacemaker would be inhibited as long as the patient's intrinsic rate was 60 beats a minute or greater. However, when the pacemaker started to pace, it would pace at 70 ppm.

ICHD Intersociety Commission for Heart Disease Resources (ICHD), the organization which came up with the first pacemaker code.

impedance In pacing, anything that opposes the normal flow of current.

intercalated disk A special material sandwiched between cardiac cells that allows for the rapid passage of electrical energy between cells; also called gap junctions.

intracardiac electrogram (IEGM) A tracing of the heart's electrical activity taken from within the heart. It contrasts with a surface ECG, which uses electrical measurements taken from the skin's surface. Pacemakers deliver IEGMs to the programmer. An IEGM is what the pacemaker "sees" and may be more useful in assessing pacing behavior than a surface ECG.

ion A charged particle which flows in and out of the semi-permeable cardiac cell membranes and changes polarization. Ions can be positively charged (cation) or negatively charged (anion).

IS-1 An abbreviation for International Standard 1, a lead and connector standardized size that accommodates leads with a 3.2 mm diameter pin. IS-1 leads and pulse generator connectors are the most commonly used in the world today.

J lead A special type of lead for use in the right atrium with a characteristic J-shape at the distal end.

lead The insulated wire that connects to the pulse generator and fixates in the patient's heart, where it can sense intrinsic activity and deliver output pulses.

left bundle branch block A conduction disorder which affects both the left anterior and left posterior fascicles in the heart. Often abbreviated LBBB, it often appears on the ECG as a notched QRS complex.

longevity The service life of a pacemaker. Since longevity is impacted by many factors, including the percentage of time paced, the output settings, and other variables, most manufacturers project estimated longevity figures for products. In clinical practice, actual device longevity will vary significantly among patients.

lower rate limit See **base rate**.

magnet behavior See **magnet mode**.

magnet mode A specially defined type of pacemaker behavior that occurs whenever a magnet is applied over the implanted pulse generator (causing the reed switch to close). Magnet mode varies by device, but generally disables most advanced features and may involve fixed-rate, asynchronous pacing. Also known as magnet behavior.

maximum tracking rate (MTR or max track) The "speed limit" on the pacemaker, the rate over which it will not allow the ventricles to be paced in response to sensed atrial activity.

membrane potential The electrical potential of cardiac cells, measured in millivolts (thousandths of a volt). Changes in membrane potential cause cardiac contractions and relaxation.

millisecond One-thousandth of one second, a very common unit of time used in pacing timing cycles. Abbreviated ms.

minute ventilation A sensor system used in rate-responsive pacemakers which detects respiration rates (based on chest movements) and adjusts the pacing rate in response to sensed need.

Mobitz I See Type I heart block.

Mobtiz II See Type II heart block.

mode switching A special feature of many dual-chamber pacemakers which allows the device to change modes in the presence of rapid, intrinsic atrial activity. Essentially, mode switching "turns off" the atrial channel of a dual-chamber pacemaker during periods of very high-rate, intrinsic atrial activity. Sometimes called **automatic mode switching (AMS)**.

MP35N A type of nickel alloy frequently used in conductor wires of pacing leads.

multisite pacing Device-based therapy which involves pacing and sensing both the right and left atria (multisite atrial pacing) or the right and left ventricles (sometimes called biventricular pacing).

myocardial cells Specialized cells in the heart muscle that possess contractility, allowing them to contract and relax.

myocardial leads A type of pacing lead designed to be attached to the outside of the heart, either by screwing into the heart's exterior or suturing on a patch. Myocardial leads, also known as epicardial leads, require a thoracotomy for implantation and are used today only in special applications.

myopotential Muscle noise which is sometimes picked up by the pacemaker's sense amplifiers and inappropriately interpreted as cardiac activity.

NASPE North American Society for Pacing and Electrophysiology, see **HRS.**

NBG code The official shorthand code that identifies pacemakers by the highest mode they can achieve and which is also widely used in clinical situations to describe programmable pacing modes. The code involves at least three and up to five letters that describe various pacemaker functions and features.

neurocardiogenic syncope A broad term for several conditions in which a neural reflex triggers systemic hypotension, characterized by both bradycardia and peripheral vasodilation. A common type of neurocardiogenic syncope is vasovagal syncope.

Ohm's law The law of electricity which states that $V = IR$, where V is voltage, I is current, and R is resistance (or impedance).

output pulse The electrical energy generated by the pacemaker and delivered to the heart. This output pulse is defined by pulse amplitude (voltage) and pulse duration (length of time, measured in milliseconds).

overdrive suppression The quality of cardiac cells which allows only one electrical impulse to travel on a pathway at any given time; this means that the first impulse to enter the pathway (from the SA node, for example) takes control of the heart and suppresses other electrical impulses which might

occur later. Overdrive suppression can be physiological (for example, the SA node is the healthy heart's dominant pacemaker because it suppresses escape rhythms) or a pacemaker algorithm (atrial pacing can overdrive the atrium).

oversensing A common sensing problem in pacing in which the pacemaker senses signals inappropriately. This causes the pacemaker to "see" intrinsic events that may not be there and to withhold pacing inappropriately. Oversensing typically leads to underpacing and shows up on the ECG in the form of long pauses.

pacemaker The implantable, low-voltage electric device for management of symptomatic bradycardias and other conduction disorders. Technically, pacemaker refers to the pulse generator and the lead(s) but sometimes it is used to refer to the pulse generator alone.

pacemaker-mediated tachycardia (PMT) A rapid ventricular rate facilitated by the presence of a pacemaker. A PMT is not caused by the pacemaker, but once a reentry tachycardia gets started, the pacemaker acts like a reentry path.

pacemaker Wenckebach A type of upper rate response in which the PV delay gets longer and longer until one of the P-waves falls into the PVARP and is not matched with a ventricular event. Also called **pseudo-Wenckebach.**

pacing interval The amount of time between paced events stated in milliseconds. When a clinician programs a pacemaker to pace at 60 pulses per minute, the pacing interval is 1000 ms.

pacing system analyzer (PSA) A small, hand-held device that can be used to gather intra-operative measurements of the pacing system.

pacing threshold The minimum amount of energy required to reliably capture (cause depolarization of) the heart. Sometimes called **stimulation threshold** or **capture threshold**.

parallel-wound coils A type of bipolar lead construction in which two conductors are individually insulated but then wrapped together in one coil.

passive filling of the ventricles The period in every cardiac cycle when the heart is completely at rest, the valves are open, and blood flows into the heart, where it collects in the lower chambers.

passive-fixation lead A lead with a fixation mechanism on the distal end that works by lodging itself in the trabeculae of the heart; examples of passive-fixation mechanisms are tines (most common) and fins.

PMT termination algorithm A special feature (or features) in some pacemakers to help prevent or break pacemaker-mediated tachycardias.

pocket The site where the pulse generator is implanted, typically in the upper chest on the patient's non-dominant side. An incision is made deep enough to reach the pectoralis fascia about an inch below and parallel to the clavicle.

polarization The predictable flow pattern of charged ions in an electrical system. In pacing, polarization is frequently observed around the electrode on a pacing lead.

port A place in the pulse generator header into which a lead may be plugged. Single-chamber pulse generators have one port, dual-chamber pulse generators have two ports, and biventricular stimulation devices may have three ports.

programmer A proprietary, tabletop computer system that is used for telemetry with the implanted pacemaker.

pseudo-Wenckebach See **pacemaker Wenckebach.**

pulse amplitude A programmable pacemaker setting which helps define the output pulse of the pacemaker. The pulse amplitude is set in volts; increasing pulse amplitude can be an efficient way to increase output pulse energy.

pulse duration See **pulse width.**

pulse generator The actual electronic device, implanted in the chest, that generates the electrical pulses that can pace the heart. Although this unit is often called the pacemaker, the pacemaker is actually the pulse generator plus lead(s).

pulse width A programmable pacemaker setting which helps define the output pulse of the pacemaker. It is set in milliseconds and determines how long a particular voltage output is delivered. Sometimes called **pulse duration.**

Purkinje fibers A very fine network of cells in the lower portion of the ventricles that conduct electricity; the Purkinje fibers are the last portion of the electrical pathway through the heart.

PV delay The timing cycle in dual-chamber pacemakers following a sensed atrial event. If the PV delay expires before an intrinsic ventricular event is sensed, then a ventricular output is delivered. Typically, the PV delay should be slightly shorter (around 25 ms) than the AV delay.

PVARP Post-ventricular atrial refractory period, a dual-chamber timing cycle on the atrial channel initiated by a ventricular event.

rate drop response A special feature in some advanced dual-chamber pacemakers which may be useful for patients with neurocardiogenic syncope. The pacemaker is programmed to a somewhat high hysteresis rate, so that pacing is mainly inhibited; should a syncopal spell occur and the patient's intrinsic rate decrease markedly, pacing commences at a higher-than-normal rate in an effort to help compensate for the temporarily diminished cardiac output.

rate adaptation See rate response.

rate modulation See rate response.

rate response A feature in modern pacemakers that allows them to respond to metabolic need by using a sensor, commonly an activity or minute ventilation sensor. Also called **rate modulation** or **rate adaptation.**

rate-responsive AV delay (RRAVD) A timing cycle in dual-chamber pacemakers that automatically shortens the AV delay in response to higher atrial rates. Often used with rate-responsive systems, RRAVD can also be useful for patients with high intrinsic atrial rates.

reed switch A small reed-like metal component within the pulse generator which can close to create an electrical circuit that causes the pacemaker to revert to magnet mode.

reentry circuit An aberrant conduction pathway in the heart which creates an endless loop for electrical impulses and results in tachycardia.

refractory period A defined period of time (usually measured in milliseconds) during which the heart will not contract. A refractory period may be physiological or it may be part of a pacemaker timing cycle. This is further subdivided into absolute refractory period, when a contraction is impossible, and a relative refractory period, when there is limited response.

repolarization Cardiac relaxation caused by a cellular response in which cell's change polarization (electrical) value. Individual cardiac cells repolarize and the heart itself can be said to repolarize (relax).

resting membrane potential The electrical potential in cardiac cells in its polarized or resting state. Every cardiac cycle returns the cells to their resting membrane potential.

rheobase On the strength–duration curve, the point at which the curve flattens. In setting output parameters, some voltage settings can be made to capture the heart if they are of sufficiently long duration. However, there is a point at which extending the pulse duration becomes moot; for example, for many patients, pacing the heart at a 0.25 V will not capture the heart, even if the pulse duration was a second long. The point at which extending the pulse duration no longer matters is the rheobase.

RV pacing Right-ventricular pacing or pacing with a lead placed in the right-ventricular apex or right-ventricular outflow tract. RV pacing can occur in single-chamber and dual-chamber modes. A great deal of unnecessary RV pacing in patients with left-ventricular dysfunction is thought to worsen heart failure (DAVID study).

safety margin An increment used to program output settings for a pacemaker in which the pacing threshold is increased. A safety margin assures capture, even with changes in pacing threshold over the course of the day or longer-term. A commonly used safety margin involves finding the pacing threshold and doubling the voltage setting.

Seldinger technique When implanting pacemakers, a venous access method that involves finding the subclavian vein using a needle rather than venous cut-down. Also called "blind subclavian stick."

sensing The ability of the pacemaker to "see" and respond to intrinsic signals. Sensing problems can often be corrected by adjusting the device's sensitivity setting.

sensor A component in certain pacemakers which allows it to detect a variable that can influence its pacing rate, for example, an activity sensor or a temperature sensor.

sensitivity A programmable pacing parameter which regulates the filter of the pacemaker. Increasing the millivolts setting decreases sensitivity, while decreasing the millivolts setting increases sensitivity.

set-screws A connection mechanism in the pulse generator connector top which helps secure the leads firmly in place. Set-screws are tightened with a small torque wrench included in the pulse generator box.

sick sinus syndrome A broad general term for any bradycardia which is caused by the fact that the sinoatrial (SA) node releases its electrical impulses too slowly, too erratically, or in extreme cases, not at all. Types of sick sinus syndrome (SSS) include sinus bradycardia, sinus arrest and silent atria.

single-chamber pacemaker A pacemaker which paces and senses only in one chamber of the heart, usually the ventricle. A single-chamber pacemaker has just one lead.

sinoatrial (SA) node A collection of highly specialized cells on the high right atrium which can spontaneously generate electricity; the SA node is sometimes called the heart's natural pacemaker.

slow calcium-sodium channels Special outlets in cardiac electrical cells which do not allow sodium or calcium to enter or exit rapidly, thus delaying electrical conduction. The cells of the AV node have slow sodium channels.

spike A common slang term for the artifact on the ECG produced by the pacemaker's output pulse.

Starling's law of contractility A scientific principle which holds that the vigor of a cardiac contraction is directly related to how much the myocardial cells are stretched. The more the cells are stretched, the more vigorously they will contract.

steroid-eluting lead A type of pacing lead with a small plug of steroid (typically dexamethasone sodium phosphate) on the distal end. This steroid reduces inflammation at the lead–tissue interface and has been associated with lower pacing thresholds and the reduction of a sharp acute-to-chronic threshold change.

stimulation threshold See pacing threshold.

strength–duration curve A chart which plots the various voltage settings (pulse amplitude) in relationship to millisecond settings (pulse width) that capture the heart in a given patient. The strength–duration curve has a characteristic shape.

stylet A thin, flexible wire that can be inserted into a pacing lead to give it enough firmness so that it can be easily maneuvered through the vasculature and into place in the heart. Stylets are sometimes offered in several degrees of stiffness.

supraventricular tachycardia A tachycardia that originates above (supra) the ventricles, typically in the atrium. A supraventricular tachycardia

(SVT) may have serious ventricular consequences, in that the rapid atrial rate may provoke a rapid ventricular response.

synchronous pacing A type of pacing (VVI, AAI, DDI, DDD, etc.) in which the pacemaker times its output pulses with the heart's own intrinsic events.

syncope Dizziness and lightheadedness which results in transient loss of consciousness. Syncope is a common symptom of rhythm disorders, but also of other conditions.

tachycardia Any number of heart rhythms in which the heart beats too quickly. Tachycardias are often named for their point of origin (atrial tachycardia, ventricular tachycardia). Tachycardias are potentially dangerous rhythm disorders. The most deadly rhythm disorder is ventricular fibrillation, a form of tachycardia.

TARP Total atrial refractory period or the PVARP + PV delay. TARP is not directly programmable, but can be adjusted by modifying the PVARP or PV delay setting.

threshold potential The point at which fast sodium channels in cardiac electrical cells open, allowing a sudden influx of positive sodium ions into the cell and causing myocardial cells to depolarize and contract.

torque wrench A special, small type of tool included in the pulse generator box used to tighten set-screws to secure the lead firmly into place in the pulse generator connector.

transvenous lead A pacing or other lead which is inserted into the vein and then maneuvered through ("trans") the vein into place in the heart.

triggered pacing A type of pacing (VVT, AAT) in which a sensed event causes an output pulse to be delivered. Triggered modes are used only for special situations or tests.

Type I heart block A form of second-degree AV block characterized by a progressive prolongation of the PR interval before a blocked beat, usually with a narrow QRS complex. It differs from first-degree AV block in that the first-degree AV block has a prolonged but stable PR duration. Also known as Mobitz I or sometimes Mobitz Type I.

Type II heart block A form of second-degree AV block characterized by a stable PR interval and a periodic "missing" QRS complex, that is, a P-wave with no associated QRS complex. The QRS complex may be wide or narrow and the missing QRS complex may occur intermittently or appear in a regular pattern (2:1, for example). Also known as Mobitz II or sometimes Mobitz Type II.

undersensing A common sensing problem in pacing in which the pacemaker inappropriately fails to sense signals it ought to see. This causes the pacemaker to pace even when it should be inhibited. Undersensing typically leads to overpacing and shows up on the ECG in the form of intrinsic events along with regular, paced activity.

unipolar Any pacing lead which has only one electrode on the distal end of the lead or any pulse generator which can accommodate such leads. For such pacemakers, the pacemaker can itself acts as the other "electrode" to complete the circuit.

upper rate behavior The way a dual-chamber pacemaker will perform when trying to deal with a high intrinsic atrial rate. If the intrinsic atrial rate exceeds the MTR and the TARP value, then pacemaker multiblock will occur. If the atrial rate exceeds the MTR but not the TARP value, then pacemaker Wenckebach will occur. Pacemaker Wenckebach is preferred over multiblock.

vasovagal syncope A type of neurocardiogenic syncope triggered by a vasodepressor reaction which causes systemic hypotension, peripheral vasodilation, nausea, photosensitivity, and sometimes bradycardia. About a quarter of all neurocardiogenic syncopal episodes are estimated to be cases of vasovagal syncope.

vena cava The largest veins in the body, which deliver de-oxygentated blood from the body back to the heart. There is a superior vena cava (the vein above the heart) and an inferior vena cava (below the heart).

ventricles The two lower, larger chambers of the heart responsible for most of the heart's pumping action.

ventricular diastole The period in every cardiac cycle when the ventricles relax.

ventricular systole The period in every cardiac cycle when the ventricles contract and pump blood.

VS-1 An abbreviation for Voluntary Standard 1, an older standard for lead and pulse generator connectors. Two main variations on VS-1 exist: VS-1A (for leads without sealing rings) and VS-1B for leads with sealing rings.

Index

Printed and bound by CPI Group (UK) Ltd, Croydon, CR0 4YY

27/10/2024

14580203-0004